Breastfeeding Your Baby

Breastfeeding Your Baby

Jane Moody, Jane Britten
and Karen Hogg

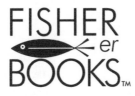

FISHER
er
BOOKS™

Publishers:	Howard W. Fisher
	Bill Fisher
	Helen V. Fisher

Managing Editor:	Sarah Trotta
North American	
Editor:	Margaret Martin, M.P.H.
Book Production:	Deanie Wood
Illustrations:	Mike Edwards, Pete Welford, Jo Dennis.
Cover Design:	FifthStreetdesign
Cover Photo:	PhotoDisc™

Published by Fisher Books, LLC
5225 W. Massingale Road
Tucson, Arizona 85743-8416
(520) 744-6110

Printed in U.S.A.
Printing 10 9 8 7 6

First published in Great Britain in 1996 as *Breastfeeding Your Baby*.

© 1996, 1997 NCT Publishing Ltd.
North American edition © 1997 Fisher Books.

Photo acknowledgments
Camilla Jessel, cover; Joanne O'Brien, xii; The National Childbirth Trust, pp. 20, 42, 58, 146; Michael Bassett, pp. 86, 98, 208; David Muscroft, p. 110; Julian Cotton Photo Library, pp. 128, 162; Egnell Ameda, p. 188.

Library of Congress Cataloging-in-Publication Data
Moody, Jane, 1954-
    Breastfeeding your baby / Jane Moody, Jane Britten, and Karen Hogg.
       p.   cm. — (National Childbirth Trust guide)
    ISBN 1-55561-122-2
    1. Breast feeding—Popular works.   I. Britten, Jane, 1950- .
II. Hogg, Karen, 1951-   . III. Title. IV. Series.
RJ216.M576   1996
649'.33—dc21

96-37910
CIP

Contents

Publisher's Note

All comments and personal accounts were given to us in confidence, so out of respect for our contributors' privacy we have changed all the names.

We have endeavored where possible to reproduce quotations verbatim, but where editing has been applied, the integrity of the quotation has been maintained.

Acknowledgments

First and most important, thank you to all the mothers who wrote about their personal experience of breastfeeding, for their courage in telling us their stories, even when it was painful to do so, and for their keenness to share their enjoyment of breastfeeding with other mothers. This book would not exist without them.

We owe a huge debt of thanks to our families, who encouraged us in this project. In particular, our husbands, who helped when word processors refused to cooperate and listened when we needed them.

Thank you to Sally Inch for allowing us first use of her table; to Ruth Dumbreck for checking our information on the Baby Friendly Hospital Initiative; to Patricia Donnithorne, NCT Information Officer, for her swift and efficient response for photocopies and references; to Sheila Perkins for her very positive support; to Rayanne O'Neill and Connie for their "first 14 days"; and to Rona McCandish and Mary Smale for reading the draft so diligently.

This book is dedicated to Stuart and Robbie Coleman; Adrienne, Matthew, Victoria and Philippa Hogg; Ruth and Thomas Moody—who began our interest in breastfeeding.

Introduction

"Feeding my son has got to be one of my greatest achievements ever and the most fulfilling experience of my life."

This book began as a leaflet and grew—the volume of information and personal stories grew so large that it could not possibly be contained in one leaflet. The leaflet was to be called *Women's Experiences of Breastfeeding,* and our book has taken that theme and expanded it. Nearly 200 women have contributed their personal experiences of breastfeeding, either for the original leaflet or specifically for our book. We owe them all a tremendous debt of gratitude for their frankness, their detailed responses and their enthusiasm for passing on their wisdom. "Feeding Files" give you information to help you with the practicalities of breastfeeding. "Background Notes" give you the facts.

We hope that the experiences of these women will give a picture of the real-life world of breastfeeding in the 1990s. We do not promise that it will all be easy if you read these pages; we do hope that if you are approaching becoming a parent, or if you are a breastfeeding mother, you will find someone here who echoes your thoughts and feelings. We do not aim to tell you how to "do" breastfeeding, although we hope you will find most of the information you need within these pages. We also hope that we have included helpful suggestions and background information to help you make your own choices.

This is an exciting time for breastfeeding. Many hospitals are taking up the challenge of becoming Baby Friendly, and many more are realizing that, up to now, there has been a gap between saying that breastfeeding is best—for you and for your baby—and providing good-quality, practical help and positive support and encouragement once your baby is born. It is into this gap that many mothers have fallen in the past. They know that they want to breastfeed, and often have a very detailed knowledge of how it should work. However, they have found that this has not been enough to enable them to succeed.

Our book follows your experience of breastfeeding through your experiences as a first-time mother—in the hospital and at home—to your growing confidence as a breastfeeding mother. We look at introducing other foods to your baby and consider some views on how long breastfeeding should last. We take you through thinking about another baby and how to manage breastfeeding a baby while coping with a toddler, and what your experience might be if you are expecting twins.

We look in some detail at various problems and difficulties which you might come across, and offer helpful information and suggestions for coping with and overcoming them, without giving up breastfeeding. We also look at some special experiences for both mother and baby. We explore the considerations around going back to work and continuing breastfeeding; and finally look at issues involved in stopping breastfeeding.

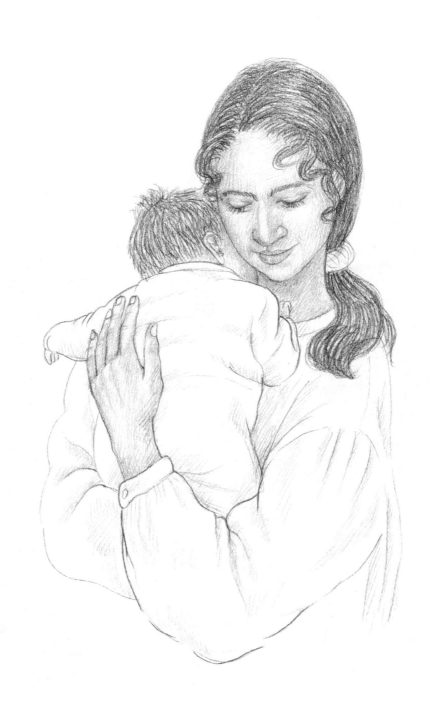

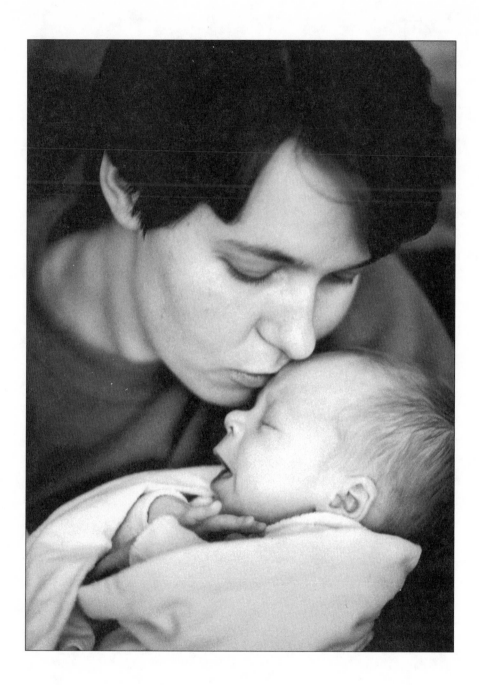

CHAPTER 1   *Before*
                    You Begin

Breastfeeding is an emotional subject. It is hard not to react when you hear the word. It involves a strong emotional response from the mother, who may be pregnant and thinking about feeding her baby. Doctors, nurses, and midwives who care for her may have their own experiences, which color their responses. The woman's family may have equally strong views.

Our responses are conditioned by our culture. In Western society, breasts mean sex, not baby-feeding. This confusion of roles leads to stress for some women, and definite rejection for others. By the time they are pregnant, most women have decided whether or not to breastfeed, even if they have not consciously thought about it.[1]

First Thoughts about Breastfeeding

Breastfeeding is almost a lost art. Today, most of us have memories of seeing babies drinking from a bottle. The images come from everywhere: television, newspapers, even children's dolls, which often come with a bottle full of 'milk.' Tip the bottle and the 'milk' disappears. It is hard to avoid the bottle-feeding culture. Breastfeeding has become something that is talked about, sometimes, but seen less often.

Memories of breastfeeding seen in childhood are scarce. The images that remain are often vivid, though, as Clare explains: *"I had few experiences of breastfeeding until I reached childbearing age. Most people I spoke to had tried to breastfeed and had not succeeded due to 'pain' and 'lack of milk' or 'not good enough milk.' My mother had tried to breastfeed me. But in the '60s her doctor told her, 'Modern women don't need to put up with all that.' It was only my grandmother, who had breastfed three children, who had the foresight to believe that women would once again realize the many benefits of breastfeeding."*

Patricia stuck firmly to her earliest impressions of how breastfeeding would be: *"I remember hearing discussions about bottle-feeding: how convenient it was, how 'civilized' and simple. But I always thought I'd breastfeed my children. I didn't want to share the feeding with anyone. As a child, I suppose I had a very idealized picture of having a baby— just sitting around all day cuddling!"*

Ellen's first conscious memory of breastfeeding was when she was about 12: *"A family friend, Sally, was breastfeeding her daughter. It was a talking point. I think there were mixed opinions about it. Some people were pleased to see a young mother succeed with breastfeeding. Some thought it was weird and hippie-ish in a conservative rural area. Funny how opinions go in circles—how natural breastfeeding can be seen as 'weird,' and artificial feeding seen as 'normal.' I spent a lot of time with the family, baby-sitting and everything. My younger sister is also a successful breastfeeder and supporter. Maybe Sally deserves our thanks for setting a good example."*

When a woman has seen a mother breastfeeding her baby, the picture often remains with her. It can affect how she feels about feeding her own babies.

Felicity's earliest memory of seeing a mother breastfeed her baby was a peaceful one. When she was about 13, she went on a country hike with her local youth group: *"One of the leaders had recently had a baby. When we stopped for a break, she sat under a nearby tree, slightly away from the bustle of the energetic teenagers, and breastfed her baby. It was a beautiful scene, with the sun filtering down through the leaves. I remember being fascinated by the mother and baby at peace with one another, despite the noise and excitement around them. Although I don't recall thinking at the time, 'When I have children, I will breastfeed them,' I believe that event must have had some positive influence on me. I can clearly remember it nearly 20 years later."*

Mothers can be influential in forming a woman's attitude to breastfeeding. If a woman was herself breastfed, she is more likely to breastfeed her own children,[1] as Jennifer affirms: *"Before I had Richard, I had no doubt about breastfeeding. It was the only thing to do. I never considered bottle-feeding as an option. This was probably due to a discussion years ago with my mom. I can't even remember how it came up. But I remember her telling me all three of us were breastfed. She was very proud of it, because a lot of moms had 'stuck their babies on the bottle and that's why there are so many fat kids around now.' I'm not sure where she got the evidence for the latter part of her statement. But it left me with a lasting impression that breast milk was IT."*

Elaine remembers her mom nursing her younger brother: *"I was nearly three at the time—she nursed Mark for about a year. I also remember my mom's Dutch friend breastfeeding her baby, which was when I was seven. I was intrigued and felt comfortable sitting with them. Breastfeeding seemed the most natural thing for her to be doing. When I was 10, my mom had my younger sister . . . and she breastfed Amy for 18 months. I used to help her get things done while she was nursing."*

For Jane, a nurse-midwife, memories of baby-feeding in her workplace are strong. The practices she describes are fairly typical of the 1970s. There are still 'hangovers' from this strict routine in some of today's hospitals: *"I worked on two wards where scheduled feeding was the rule. Feeding was every four hours for two or three minutes on each side, increasing daily. No feeding at all for the first six hours except dextrose! I didn't realize how strange this was. But I can't remember being concerned about babies crying. There were plenty of other things that horrified me. At night, the babies were all kept in the nursery and fed—on evaporated milk—even when asked expressly not to. The moms just weren't told about it. It used to be called white dextrose!*

"My lasting memory of the babies was how sleepy and 'good' they were. We woke them up four hours after the start of their last feeding, changed their diapers and gave them a bottle (most were bottle-fed). If they weren't drinking fast enough, the hole [in the nipple] was enlarged. The feeding had to be finished within 20 minutes. Diaper changing took 10 minutes. And the babies were put back in their cribs to sleep until their next feeding. It all seemed so ordered and simple. How great was the contrast when Katy was born!

"Just before Katy was born, I read Breast Is Best, *by the Stanways. The book was revolutionary to me then. It was so positive and encouraging. Breastfeeding became much more complex and interesting. The idea of demand feeding, with mother and baby communicating, was wonderful. Just the idea that your baby can be able and allowed to set the pace for feeding was completely new. In contrast with some hospitals—where the baby is treated as the 'enemy,' forced to conform to a set of rules—to be allowed and encouraged to respond to my baby's needs as the Stanways suggested was wonderful."*

Deciding to Breastfeed

Women give many reasons for their decision to breastfeed. The most common are that breastfeeding is best for the baby, it will be convenient, and that it will lead to a closer bond between mother and baby.[1]

Shawna was determined to breastfeed her first baby: *"With a history of asthma and eczema myself, having read about this subject, I knew my child would have a greater chance of not inheriting these problems if she was breastfed."*

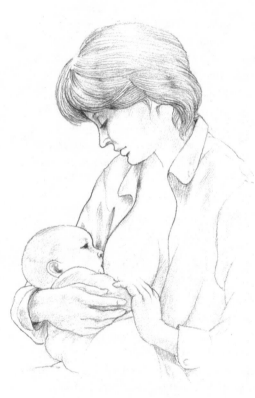

Amy recalls being curious about breastfeeding: *"I was aware that my brother and I had been bottle-fed. I also remember my aunt having her first child and being so ill with asthma after a Cesarean that she couldn't breastfeed. She had wanted to. She was taking the child overseas to live and knew that it was both cheaper and safer to breastfeed. So I had only really seen women bottle-feeding. At the same time, I knew that breastfeeding was considered the best option. So when I had Timothy and was asked how I was going to feed, I chose to breastfeed. I never really looked for support or information on the subject. I thought all I had to do was choose."*

BACKGROUND NOTES

Choices

In 1990, a survey was made of infant feeding in England.[1] Mothers were asked how they chose to feed their babies, and to give their reasons.

Choosing breastfeeding

- Breastfeeding is best for the baby. This reason was given by 82% of mothers.

- Breastfeeding is more convenient—no bottles to prepare and no sterilizing. Thirty-six percent of mothers thought this was important.

- Bonding between mother and baby was thought to be better when the baby is breastfed by 23% of mothers.

- Breastfeeding is cheaper than bottle-feeding. This was given as a reason for breastfeeding by 17% of mothers.

- Among mothers who have breastfed a child, 29% gave their previous experience as a reason for breast-feeding again.

- Breastfeeding is natural. Fourteen percent felt this was important.

- Breastfeeding is best for the mother too. Eight percent of mothers gave this as a reason for breastfeeding.

- Other reasons given by small numbers of women include the influence of doctors, nurses, friends or relatives.

- If a woman was herself breastfed, she is much more likely to want to breastfeed. Three-fourths of women who were breastfed chose to breast-feed their own babies. 70% of women who were both breast and bottle-fed also chose breastfeeding, as did 48% of those who had been bottle-fed themselves.

- If a mother's friends breastfeed, this is also an influence. Eighty-four percent of women who said that most of their friends breastfed, planned to do the same.

Choosing bottle-feeding

- Other people can feed the baby. This was the most important reason for bottle-feeding for 39% of the women who were surveyed.

- Among mothers who had previously bottle-fed, 39% chose to do so again.

- The idea of breastfeeding was not liked by 21% of mothers. Another 7% felt it was too embarrassing.

- Seeing how much milk the baby has taken was a reason for choosing the bottle for 6% of mothers.

- Medical reasons were given for bottle-feeding by 3% of mothers.

- Returning to work soon after the birth was a reason for bottle-feeding for 5% of mothers.

- Among other reasons given by small numbers of women, 1% reported having been persuaded to bottle-feed by other people.

- If most of a mother's friends bottle-feed, 54% of women also choose to bottle-feed.

- Mothers who were themselves bottle-fed are more likely to do the same. Slightly more than half of the women surveyed who were bottle-fed planned to feed their baby this way.

BACKGROUND NOTES

What's special about breast milk?

Breast milk is a living fluid. It is made by you just for your baby. So it is the most special food there is. No other product can ever come close. It is not possible to list everything in breast milk. Each new piece of research into this amazing fluid uncovers another vital ingredient babies need for their development and growth.

Colostrum

Colostrum is extra-special. It is the fluid in a mother's breasts at the time her baby is born, before her true milk comes in. It is rich in protein, immune factors, vitamins, anti-infectious agents, living cells and minerals. Colostrum protects the newborn baby until his own immune system begins to function. Colostrum helps his digestive system begin to function well. It contains all the nutrients he needs.

The basic nutrients in breast milk

- *Protein* Protein is needed for growth. Human babies are meant to grow slowly and be fed often. That's why just a small part of human milk is protein: about 1%. Protein breaks down into curds (casein) and whey. Breast milk is largely whey. Cow's milk contains much more casein. Breast milk has no lactoglobulin. This part of cow's-milk protein, which is also found in some infant formulas, is believed to cause allergic reactions in some babies.

- *Carbohydrate* Most of the carbohydrate in breast milk is lactose (milk sugar). Lactose is important for brain growth. The baby's brain is large and grows rapidly.

- *Fat* Fat is needed to provide energy (calories). The fat in breast milk digests well, with almost no waste. Essential long-chain fatty acids in breast milk are important for the growth and development of the baby's brain. These fatty acids are not naturally present in cow's milk or infant formula. Formula makers may include some of these essential fats in their products in the future. But at this time no formulas sold in the United States or Canada contain these essential fatty acids.

- *Water* Breast milk contains all the water a baby needs. Even in extreme heat or fever, a breastfed baby needs no extra water.

- *Vitamins* Almost all women are able to provide all the vitamins their babies need in their breast milk. A woman would have to be very obviously deficient in a vitamin for the levels in her breast milk to be less than adequate.

- *Minerals* Although the iron content of breast milk is low, it is absorbed 20 times better than the iron in formula milk. Other minerals are present in ideal balances for the baby.

Added extras

This is where breast milk really scores over infant formula. Breast milk contains many "nonnutritive" factors that help protect and nurture the baby in his first few months. Immune factors help protect the baby until his own immune system has developed. Living cells, such as white cells, fight infection. Hormones and enzymes are present, too. All these add up to a truly unique food that cannot be copied. Each mother produces the perfect food for *her* baby.

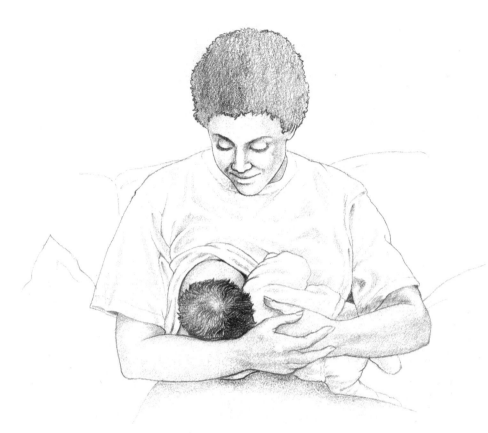

The feelings that underlie women's decisions to breastfeed vary great-
ly. Some women may feel anxious and lack confidence. This may be
reinforced if their mothers or close friends did not breastfeed successfully. Others may be optimistic and self-assured, boosted by a supportive partner or friends with positive breastfeeding experiences. You
may come to breastfeeding "determined to succeed." Or you may plan
to "give it a try and see what happens." As Liz found, family influences
are strong: *"Before my son was born, I tried not to have any fixed ideas
about anything I was going to do during or after the birth. But I was
very eager to breastfeed my baby. I was a little concerned, because my
mother had not been very successful at nursing me, my sister or my
brother. But I was encouraged by my sister, who breastfed her son and
then her daughter, born only six weeks before my son."*

When Ruth trained as a hospital-nursery nurse, breastfeeding was promoted. But her attitude changed when she spent two weeks on a
maternity ward: *"For the first time, I became aware of problems women*

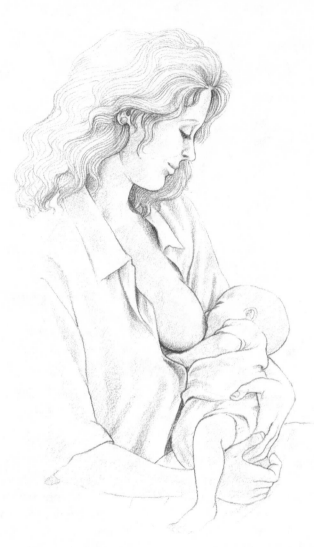

run into when breastfeeding. Most mothers were breastfeeding. And although there were hints of a possible failure, my attitude toward these women was they should still give it a try. But for the first time, I felt that there could be problems.

"Later on, I worked in the nursery exclusively. Sterilizing and making up bottles was tedious. The babies' feeding patterns were all different. Some would take up to an hour to feed. These bottle-feeding experiences were valuable in reinforcing my feelings towards breastfeeding. I was sure bottle-feeding could be no easier or more convenient than breast."

Partners can be very important. It is very hard for a woman to breast-feed if her partner does not support and encourage her. One study in the United States found that strong approval by the father of breast-feeding led to a high incidence of breastfeeding (98.1%). Only 26.9% breastfed when the father didn't care how his baby was fed.[2] Both Lois and her partner come from breastfeeding backgrounds. He was breast-fed; so were his brother and sister. Her mother breastfed all four of her children: *"Soon after my husband and I learned I was pregnant, we discussed how we would feed the baby. I was glad to hear that he was strongly in favor of my breastfeeding. This encouraged me, because I knew I could count on his wholehearted support. I believe I would have been less enthusiastic about breastfeeding if he hadn't cared."*

Many women have already decided how they want to feed their baby before they become pregnant. But the health providers you meet during your pregnancy can have a significant effect on your attitude toward breastfeeding. Laura's experience was disturbing: *"At an early prenatal visit, a man in a white coat walked into the exam room. The nurse was taking my blood pressure. He did not introduce himself. I assumed he was a doctor. He glanced at my notes, and asked me if I planned to breastfeed. He squeezed my nipple really hard. Then he frowned and scribbled in his notes and walked out. I asked the nurse to explain. She said he probably thought that I would not be able to breast-feed because my nipples were very flat. When she saw my horrified expression, she suggested that I start to pull my nipples out and roll them between my fingers when having a shower. I couldn't believe I was hear-ing this! I left feeling depressed at the possibility that I would not be able to breastfeed. I brought up the subject with my family doctor. When she examined me, she said that she didn't think it was a problem a hungry baby couldn't figure out."*

Learning about Breastfeeding

Learning about breastfeeding—theory and practice—before the birth can be a way of boosting confidence. Private childbirth classes often include at least one session about breastfeeding. Hospital-run classes may also include a session, but sometimes the time is split between breast- and bottle-feeding. Although it is done frequently, teaching all mothers-to-be how to make up infant formula violates the World Health Organization (WHO) Code on the Marketing of Breast Milk Substitutes.

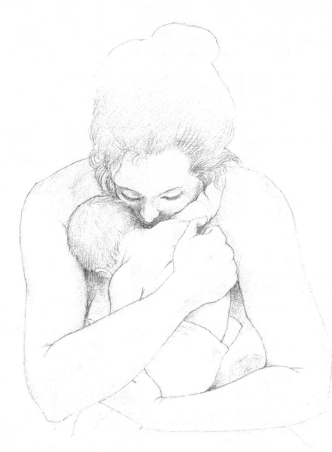

Colette attended private childbirth classes. They included a session with a breastfeeding counselor: *"I don't know that I learned much about nursing techniques at that time. I don't think you can really absorb much until you're doing it yourself. But I did gain a lot of confidence from her. She made breastfeeding seem natural and easy. Before that, all I had heard was negative—horror stories from friends."*

Libby feels she was typical of many first-timers: *"I was anxious to do 'nothing but the best.' As far as I was concerned, I was going to breastfeed my baby and that was all there was to it. I believed it was simply a matter of choice, either to breastfeed or bottle-feed. In the hospital, I had many nurses trying to get Neil latched on, but without too much success. I had to give up nursing Neil after a couple of weeks. Soon after, I felt rejected by Neil. When I learned I was pregnant with Julia, I decided I would not even try to breastfeed her. But as time went by, I thought to myself that I might try. I continued to tell doctors and midwives that*

I planned to bottle-feed, though. I wanted to be left alone in my decision, without pressure. So I read up on breastfeeding and relaxed about the whole thing. After a wonderful birth, Julia was put to my breast and nursed well right away. I was overjoyed! So was Julia—she wouldn't stop."

Rebecca found that classes were useful, if only to open her eyes about feeding a baby: *"I didn't listen during the prenatal class about 'How to prepare a bottle.' I was going to breastfeed. Why should I need to know how to sterilize and prepare bottles of formula? I thought that people who bottlefed did so because they didn't want to breastfeed. And I couldn't understand why anyone would not want to do what was best for the baby. Strangely enough, it was after a talk by a breastfeeding counselor that it first occurred to me that I might not be able to breastfeed. The counselor said that sometimes breastfeeding does not work out for some mothers and babies. That was the first inkling I had that it might be possible that I might not be able to breastfeed my baby."*

Some women, Ana included, who try to find out about breastfeeding before the birth feel that the information they get is poor or negative: *"I am currently breastfeeding my second child, now five months old. I feel very strongly there is a lack of prenatal advice about the subject. After reading and classes, I felt well-prepared for the birth itself. But I felt totally unprepared for breastfeeding. Most books I looked at were illustrated with soft-focus photographs of naked mother and child engaged in breastfeeding. Although problems, like cracked nipples and a poor milk supply, were listed, the heartache and pain of these were never described."*

Others, like Shawna, are too worried about the birth to think about what comes after it: *"I went to prenatal classes, but when it came to breast-*

feeding, I couldn't remember anything we'd been told. I remember the person giving the breastfeeding class holding a doll in her arms. I don't know if it was my lack of concentration or her inability to keep me interested that was the problem. It might have been both. I know it was very hard to see past the birth for me. I wanted so much to see my baby and make sure she or he was OK. It felt like tempting fate to spend too much time preparing for life with a normal, healthy baby until I had one. So I grabbed my breastfeeding books and leaflets and took them with me to the hospital to read after the birth."

For Moira, information was the key to success: *"I wanted as much information as I could get about establishing and continuing with breastfeeding before the baby came. I believed that this would improve my chances of breastfeeding successfully. I went to two prenatal courses. They were useful. They gave me the chance to ask questions about aspects of breastfeeding I was unsure about or didn't understand. Although some of the material in the two courses was the same, I liked hearing things said by two different people with slightly different approaches. It helped reinforce some issues I was unclear about. Also, attending two different classes put me in touch with two groups of expectant mothers. This was useful in the months that followed. The literature from these classes also helped, particularly from La Leche League. And the handouts from the breastfeeding counselor that showed good positioning of the baby at the breast were great."*

For Mother or Baby?

You may think about starting to breastfeed because you feel you should, not really expecting to enjoy it. Or you may look forward to it eagerly like Tami, for yourself as well as for the baby: *"I had been looking forward to breastfeeding. I'd learned all I could from books, midwives, and members of La Leche League and the International Childbirth Education Association. I think I'd wanted to breastfeed ever since I had watched my cousin nursing her baby when I was 10!"*

Gail put her baby first, before her own emotions: *"To be honest, I wasn't really looking forward to breastfeeding my baby. But as an ex-pediatric nurse, I knew that it was really the best start I could give. And also the cheapest—an important point, because I was giving up work and money would be tight."*

From talking to others, Angela was aware that for a number of women, their strongest reason for breastfeeding is the health of the child, rather than their own feelings. They may even continue to breastfeed despite not enjoying it: *"It wasn't like that for me. The fact that I knew it was best for her gave me extra back-up for something that I wanted to do for myself."*

Women who feel unsure about whether they will breast- or bottle-feed may find it hard to discuss their feelings because of the pressure they feel to breastfeed. Or no one may seem ready to listen to their feelings.

Elaine found the pressure to breastfeed was intense: *"I felt compelled to breastfeed. I have met other mothers who said publicly that they 'couldn't' breastfeed and privately that they simply did not want to—but also that they did not wish to admit this."*

Sometimes a policy to encourage breastfeeding can spill over into pressure, as Terri found: *"It is what your mother did. It is what the hospital made clear that you ought to do. I recall sharing my feelings* (about not wanting to breastfeed) *with my male family doctor when I was 39 weeks pregnant. His advice was simple. Breast milk was for babies, cow's milk for calves. I never really forgave him! What a shame that no one else could try and listen or understand how I felt at that time."*

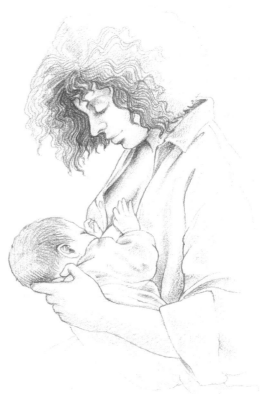

BACKGROUND NOTES

Physical changes to the breasts

The basic structure within the breasts develops at puberty. During pregnancy, the ducts (vessels down which the milk will flow) and milk-producing cells grow and multiply. The blood supply to the breasts increases. Milk begins to be made at around five months of pregnancy. You may notice very early in your pregnancy that your breasts are changing. They may become very sensitive and tender as all the rapid changes take place.

Breasts and nipples— all shapes and sizes

Breasts and nipples change during pregnancy. Generally, they become larger and the area around the nipple, the *areola,* darkens. The size of your breasts is not an important feature of breastfeeding. A woman with small breasts is just as able to produce enough milk for her baby as a woman with larger breasts.

The shape of your nipples is also not important. As far as the baby is concerned, it isn't too likely that he will ever meet or nurse from another pair of breasts. To him, his mother's breasts are just perfect.

During pregnancy or soon after birth, most women's nipples tend to stand out a little from the breast. When breastfeeding, the baby takes a large "mouthful" of your breast into his mouth. While he sucks, the nipple is drawn out more. Some nipples stand out proudly from the rest of the breast

tissue, some not so much. Others can be almost flat. And some can be turned inwards (looking like craters).

Sometimes your breasts may be viewed by a healthcare provider while you are pregnant. You may be told that your nipples are flat or inverted, and that this will make breastfeeding difficult or impossible. You may be told that you need to "prepare" your nipples for breastfeeding. Suggested treatments may include nipple-stretching exercises or wearing breast shells or shields. (Both are advertised as capable of helping the nipples stand out.) Recent research into prenatal treatments for flat or inverted nipples has shown that wearing breast shields or doing nipple exercises are *not* helpful.[3]

The researchers in this study stressed that many of the mothers with inverted nipples who entered their trial were breastfeeding well. *The baby's position at the breast is the most important factor for success—not the shape of the breast.*

Once nursing well, the baby's sucking action can and does draw out flat and inverted nipples. The nipples may stay erect after nursing. Or they may revert to their natural state. Some mothers find that their nipples remain erect after breastfeeding. Many women in this trial reported that their caregivers had discouraged them from even trying to breastfeed because of the shape of their nipples. But the modern myth, that it is not possible to breastfeed with inverted nipples, simply is not true.

Breast size and shape vary from woman to woman . . .

Your breasts will change during pregnancy . . .

and while you are breastfeeding.

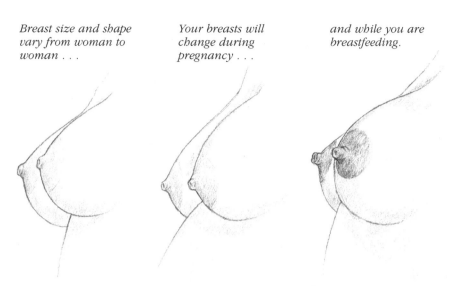

It is important to discuss your feelings with a healthcare provider who will listen to you and accept what you are saying. You should be given many opportunities for this—as many as you want. Pregnancy and early parenthood are emotional times. It will be more stressful if you feel you cannot talk freely about your feelings without being judged.

Sex during Pregnancy

Pregnancy brings changes to your breasts. These changes will affect your life as a sexual couple. In the early weeks, your nipples may be quite sensitive to touch. You may wish no contact during foreplay. Or you may prefer more stimulation. There could be concerns about miscarriage in the early months. If so, you may be advised not to have intercourse at all for a while.

As the pregnancy progresses, you will need to find positions for making love that do not squash your belly or your breasts. Sometimes these changes add excitement to your relationship, as Karen discovered: *"When I was pregnant, my husband and I enjoyed a carefree sex life. We had no contraception needs, no worries. I seemed to have an increased sex drive. And he found my changing body shape exciting and stimulating. He said that in his eyes I was the most beautiful woman in the world. And he found himself increasingly attracted to me far more often. This was wonderful and made me feel very loved and wanted."*

FEEDING FILE

Looking forward to breastfeeding together

- Attend the prenatal session on breastfeeding with your partner. Discuss how you both feel about breastfeeding. Include memories, your own experiences, negative feelings and any concerns. For example: How might your partner feel about you breastfeeding in front of male relatives or friends? And how do you feel?

- Discuss how running the household may change according to your needs as a new family.

- Talk to each other as much as you can about the changes you are going through as a pregnant woman and an expectant father. Share your thoughts (and fantasies) of life after the birth. You may learn that you have similar worries and that you are looking forward to the same joys.

- Expect major changes in your routines as a couple without children.

Prenatal Preparation

Sometimes you may be told that you need to "prepare" your nipples in some way for breastfeeding. It is not useful to "prepare" the nipples by rubbing or scrubbing them. Nipples are sensitive because they are *supposed* to be sensitive. "Toughening" them has no effect on later soreness—except perhaps to worsen it. And you don't need to express colostrum, either. It's too bad that there are still plenty of people who give this kind of advice to mothers:

"On my doctor's advice, I tried to prepare my nipples by rubbing them, first with a rough towel, later with a soft toothbrush."

"I tried scrubbing my breasts with a washcloth after reading you should in some book. I gave up after about two minutes when I felt the pain! After that I decided I'd wait and suffer when the baby was born."

Nature 'prepares' your body for birth and your breasts for breastfeeding. All you have to do is sit back and wait, and enjoy your growing, changing shape.

FEEDING FILE

Preparing for breastfeeding

Your body prepares for breastfeeding while you are pregnant. The structure of the milk ducts and milk-producing cells develops. And the blood supply to the breasts increases. Most breasts grow in size during pregnancy as a result of these changes. Some women find that, as their breasts increase in size, they feel better when they wear a supportive bra. It is good to remember, though, that the size of your breasts does not relate in any way to their capacity for producing milk.

As pregnancy progresses, colostrum begins to be made in the breasts. You may notice this creamy-colored substance on the nipples. These deposits come off when you shower or bathe. Some mothers leak enough colostrum to need to wear a breast pad. This leaking is perfectly natural. It will not "use up" your milk. Some women do not leak, but will still have colostrum in their breasts.

In the past, there was a lot of advice about ways to "toughen up" the nipples, such as scrubbing the nipples with rough towels. This isn't helpful and is very painful.

Before the birth

- Find out about breastfeeding. Clear and correct information from a good, honest source is vital. Watch out for "myths" and "old wives tales".

- Attend prenatal classes. Most hospital classes and private childbirth classes include at least one session on breastfeeding.

- Discuss breastfeeding with your doctor, midwife and other people who will care for you.

- Breastfeeding counselors (lactation consultants) and La Leche League leaders are happy to discuss breastfeeding at any time. They are trained to focus on the mother and her needs.

- Books about breastfeeding should be available at all good bookstores. La Leche League publishes leaflets and books on a number of breastfeeding topics.

- In the United States, women with low incomes can get information and support from their nearest WIC office. (WIC stands for *Women, Infants and Children*. It provides food coupons and support to women with low incomes, and their infants and children.) Call your state or county Public Health Department for the WIC office nearest you.

- In Canada, you may receive information and support from your provincial or territorial Ministry of Health. See page 225 for contact information.

- Think in advance about where you will get support and encouragement once you are breastfeeding. Talk about your decision with your family. Make sure they will support you. This can help prevent conflict when the baby is born.

BACKGROUND NOTES

Why breastfeed?

In terms of health, breastfeeding is the best, both for you and for your baby.

Tones your body

- Breastfeeding helps your body recover quickly from giving birth. Hormones released when your baby sucks contract your uterus a bit more each time you nurse. The same hormones help tone your muscles again.

- You may find that you lose weight more quickly if you breastfeed. Breastfeeding uses up the fat you stored up in pregnancy. In one study, women who breastfed for at least 6 months lost an average of 4-$\frac{1}{2}$ pounds more than nonbreastfeeders during the first year of the baby's life. The greatest loss was in the 3- to 6-month period.[5] Some women only lose weight once they have finished breastfeeding.

- Breastfeeding helps you to relax and feel calm. Once the milk starts to flow, your hormones help you to relax and enjoy it.

Rewarding and pleasant

- Breastfeeding brings you close to your baby. It can feel good: warm and comforting, to you as well as your baby.

- Many women feel intense pleasure when their baby nurses. Others feel a great sense of pride in seeing their baby grow strong and healthy on their milk alone.

- You never have to keep your baby waiting with breastfeeding. There is always milk in your breasts. And it is always ready.

Protects you naturally

- Studies show that breastfeeding your baby for three months helps protect you from breast cancer before menopause. The risk is cut in half.[6,7] It also helps to protect you from ovarian cancer.[8]

- Exclusive breastfeeding—that is, giving nothing but breast milk—can also help provide a healthy space between children, if you plan to have another child.[9,10] *But breastfeeding does not provide complete contraception.*

- If you breastfeed, you are less at risk of osteoporosis (thin or brittle bones) than if you do not.[11] Although the levels of calcium in your bones fall while you are breastfeeding, your bone mineral content is improved. And by six months after weaning your calcium levels are higher than they would be if you had not breastfed at all.

- Protection also extends to hip fractures. One study found that women who had never breastfed had twice the risk of hip fractures as women who had breastfed. The longer you breastfeed, the greater the protection. Breastfeeding for longer than nine months for each child can reduce your risk to one-fourth that of nonbreastfeeders.[12]

BACKGROUND NOTES

Ideal food for your baby

- Your body has fed and protected your baby for the last nine months. Breastfeeding is designed to do the same for the next nine months.

- Breast milk is the very best food your baby will ever have. It contains every nutrient your baby needs to grow and develop to her full potential.[13,14] It even changes as your baby grows to meet her changing needs. She needs nothing else for the first four to six months.

Best for your baby's growth

- Formula milk can copy some of the basic nutrients in breast milk. But there are properties in breast milk that cannot be copied.[16,17,18,19]

- Breast milk is uniquely designed to make sure that your baby's brain and central nervous system develop to their full potential.

- Studies have shown that breast milk is important for the correct development of babies' eyesight, especially if they are born prematurely.[20]

Important for health

- Because your milk contains antibodies, breastfeeding is important in helping your baby stay healthy.[21,22] Most important, breastfeeding protects your baby from dangerous stomach germs, which cause diarrhea. Formula-fed babies are five to 10 times more likely to get gastroenteritis than breastfed babies.[23]

- Breastfeeding also protects against breathing problems and chest infections that cause wheezing, such as bronchitis, bronchiolitis and pneumonia. Studies have found that this protection can last for years after breastfeeding has ended.[24,25]

- Babies who are strictly breastfed, with no added formula, until at least four months of age, suffer from half the number of ear infections of those who are never breastfed. They also have 40% fewer ear infections than those who receive supplements of formula.[26,27]

- Babies who are not strictly breastfed for at least two months double their risk of getting insulin-dependent diabetes.[28,29,30]

Protects against allergies

- Breastfeeding can help protect your baby from allergies such as eczema and asthma. It can also help make these allergies less severe if they do develop in your baby.[24]

- Many experts recommend that babies from families with allergies be breastfed without any supplements for at least six months, if possible.[31]

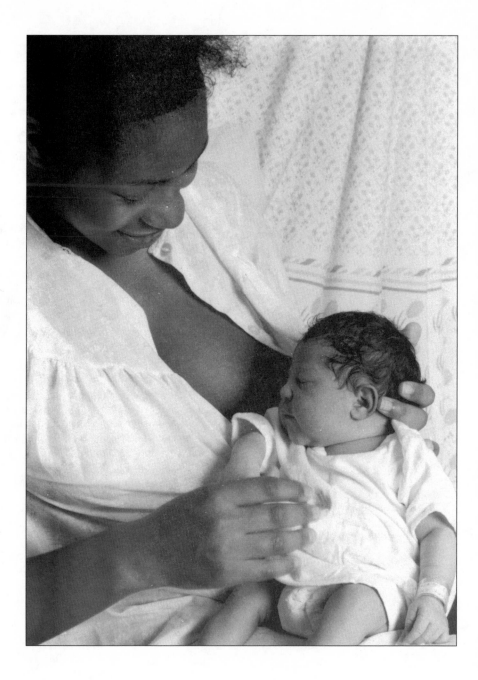

CHAPTER 2

The Early Days

Beginnings

For many mothers and babies, starting to breastfeed is problem-free and pleasant. You may find that your baby knows just how to get a good meal. All you have to do is show him where it is. Ruth's baby, Laura, was alert and nursed right away: *"This was a very positive beginning. I felt so close to my baby and very much needed. She seemed to know just what to do. She was allowed to nurse for a few minutes. And I was able to nurse her again after she'd been checked and I'd been stitched up. I felt this was a treasured and rewarding way to begin."*

Your first breastfeeding can produce very powerful feelings. It can be a sensual and fulfilling experience, unique to each mother. For some, it is almost beyond words:

"I put him to the breast within minutes of birth. He sucked for just a few seconds. With the first feeding I was surprised at the powerful physical and emotional feelings it produced." Hilary's experience was simple and followed an easy birth. But even if you have a more complicated delivery those first moments can be precious, as Lesley found out: *"The first time I put our little girl to the breast was minutes after having a C-section. Me being flat on my back, Anne was placed on my right side. My nightdress was unbuttoned. I watched as the midwife edged Anne towards me. She teased her lips to open and—bingo! Anne was latched on with such speed and accuracy. It was a bulls-eye the first time! I cannot describe my feelings of sheer joy and relief that the breastfeeding was going well. The birth had been so long and drawn out, full of problems. I had felt totally powerless. But now here was something no one else could interfere with. And the two of us were doing it perfectly—just Anne and me, close, cuddling, and both relieved."*

BACKGROUND NOTES

How breastfeeding works

There are 15 to 20 milk-producing glands in each breast. Milk is made in these glands from substances absorbed from the bloodstream and stored in the milk ducts.

Making milk

Milk will be made in the breasts whether or not you breastfeed. Once the placenta comes out, the pregnancy hormones give way to the milk-making hormone, *prolactin.* This hormone triggers the breasts to make milk. It also has a calming and relaxing effect on you.

The removal of milk from the breast is important in its continued production. There is a chemical in the milk that stops milk from being produced if it is not used. If milk stays in the breast too long, this chemical (autocrine inhibitor or "suppressor") will begin to reduce the amount of milk produced. Babies need to nurse frequently in the early weeks to prevent levels of this chemical suppressor from building up.[32]

Once the baby starts to nurse, the hormone *oxytocin* is released into the bloodstream. It reaches the breasts and contracts the muscles around the milk cells. It forces them to push the milk into the ducts. This is what some women feel as the "let-down" or milk-ejection reflex: often a warm, tingling feeling. Not all women feel this reflex, though. The absence of the sensation does not mean that the reflex is not working.

Foremilk and hindmilk

The milk the baby takes in a feeding changes during the feeding. When he first begins to suck, the baby will receive *foremilk.* This milk is watery to look at and low in fat and calories.

But it's high in the milk sugar, lactose. As the feeding progresses, *hindmilk* is released. This milk is higher in fat and calories.

Fat is very sticky. It sticks to the walls of the milk-producing cells. As the let-down squeezes the milk cells, foremilk is released first. As the feeding goes on, more fat is forced into the ducts. As the amount of milk in the breast goes down, the fat content goes up. At the end of the feeding, the fat content of the milk is very high. It is probably this quality that helps the baby decide he has had enough.

Baby-led nursing—that is, letting the baby decide when to nurse, how often and for how long—makes sure that he gets enough calories at each feeding. If he is taken off the breast before he is ready, he may not receive enough of this high-fat, high-calorie milk. If he is swapped to the other breast too soon, he will have to take all the low-fat foremilk in that breast before he gets to the calorie-rich hindmilk again. His stomach may get too full before he gets enough calories.

If the baby receives too much lowfat foremilk, he may get uncomfortable and "burpy." Foremilk is very sugary. Too much of it makes the breast milk pass through the baby's intestines too quickly. This means that the enzymes of the gut do not completely break down the breast milk, so all the valuable nutrients can't be absorbed. His diapers may often be filled with green, frothy stools, and he seems fretful and always hungry. It may help to let the baby nurse as long as he wants to from one breast. Then, if he wants to go back to the breast soon after he has finished, get him to nurse from the same breast again. The high-fat hindmilk will help slow his digestion and help him feel full.

You may wish to put your baby to the breast right after birth. This will help the placenta come out. The hormone that causes the muscles around the milk-producing cells to contract, "letting down" your milk, also makes your uterus contract.

"My second baby had nursed right away. I looked forward to this one doing the same. But there was a small problem. We had left the cord intact until it stopped pulsating. It was a very short cord. So there I was, doubled over, dangling a nipple into her mouth because she could not reach. And the cord was pulling and tweaking at me from inside. Really uncomfortable!"

There is good evidence that babies who begin breastfeeding right after birth are twice as likely to be breastfeeding at the end of two weeks as are those who begin later.[1]

"Putting the baby to the breast" does not always mean that the baby nursed. Not all babies—or mothers—are ready to nurse right away. It is not clear how much of the benefit of early contact between you and your baby comes from the contact itself—touching, feeling, smelling and looking—and how much comes from nursing.

Jill's baby did not want to nurse right away: *"After the birth of my first baby, I was a wreck. It was a very long labor with a lot of intervention— induction, epidural, forceps and episiotomy. I couldn't hold him very well. I was still attached to all sorts of machines. And I was lying down, numb from the waist down. My partner held him. Then the nurses helped me to sit up a little. I managed to hold him and look at him and touch him. I offered him my breast. He licked it and nuzzled it, but didn't really nurse."*

Sometimes there are medical reasons to delay putting the baby to the breast. You may need stitches or be recovering from an anesthetic. Or your baby may be ill or premature. It helps to know that many babies who do not nurse in the first few hours after birth do go on to breast-feed successfully and happily.

Shawna awoke from the general anesthetic (for a Cesarean section) to be told she had a healthy 9 lb. 10 oz. son: *"My less-than-enthusiastic response was, 'OK, great—my stomach hurts.' The next time I woke up, I was a little better. But I was still very drowsy. At least I could just about sit up in bed and hold Marco. I tried to nurse him. But I could not find a way to hold him near my breast and also away from my still-swollen stomach. That night, he slept in the nursery. With my permission, he was given a bottle. The next morning brought a whole new meaning to life. The pain-killing shots were working. I had slept and felt half-human. After I had a bed bath, they asked if I wanted to try to nurse my baby again. He managed his first really good feeding at about 28 hours old."*

Frances didn't breastfeed her daughter, Melanie, until she was four days old: *"I had planned to bottle-feed but she wouldn't take the bottle. So my cousin suggested I try breastfeeding. A lactation consultant came to help me. She was great. She helped me to get comfortable. I had a lot of stitches and had been very uncomfortable when bottle-feeding. Melanie nursed well at once. She took to it like a duck to water."*

You may find that your baby, like Lisa's, doesn't want to nurse in the early hours after delivery: *"I did not nurse him in the delivery room, despite my intentions. I was too dazed to get my act together. (And no one suggested I try it!) A little later, in the recovery room, I asked the nurse if I could try nursing him. 'You can if you want to,' she said, 'but we usually bring them to you after six hours for a feeding.' I tried to nurse him. But although Jack was very alert and wide-eyed for the first hour after birth, he showed no interest. The nurse did not seem bothered, so I gave up trying. We got to know each other in other ways."*

The Baby's Position Matters

Right from the start, take time to position your baby well at your breast. This will help keep you from getting sore. It will also help your baby milk the breast well. Start by getting comfortable. Find out how to hold your baby comfortably at your breast. If you have had a Cesarean birth or a lot of stitches, you may need to ask the nurse to help you. Try different positions until you find one that is comfortable.

Shawna tried everything, but success only came on the second day: *"I tried holding him with his feet tucked under my arm, lying on a pillow, but it wasn't a huge success. The nurse suggested lying down, with Marco lying next to me, either on the bed or on a pillow. This didn't work because he was too high on the pillow. And he was so long he still kicked my stitches when he was laid on the bed. We tried pillows on my stomach next, holding Marco in the crook of my arm. This was fine until he wiggled off the pillows. Later that day, I was allowed out of bed. Sitting in a chair to nurse Marco was a huge improvement. Someone found me a footstool. This, combined with about three pillows, raised Marco high enough above my stitches to be able to nurse. Once he got the hang of it, everything was fine. He had his first really good feeding at about 28 hours old and never looked back."*

Beth's first feeding was not as she would have liked it: *"I was sitting on the delivery bed feeling very sore. I had needed some stitches. I had to sit with my knees apart. I couldn't sit up straight because it hurt too*

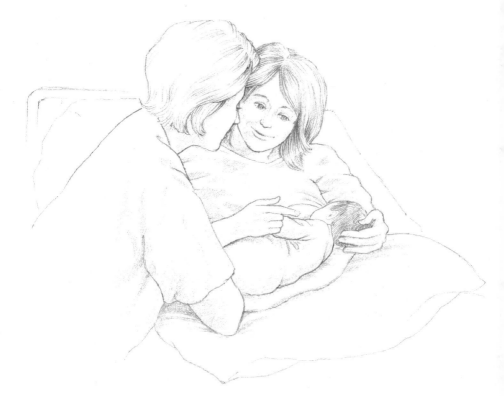

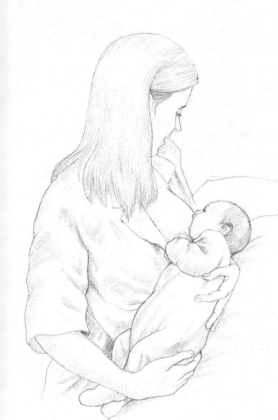

much. I really wanted to lie down, but the head of the bed was still up, so I couldn't. I felt dirty, sweaty and horrible, so I didn't feel relaxed. Besides, Emma was gazing up at me serenely, and didn't seem to be in a big hurry to nurse."

Getting your baby to latch on to the breast comes next. Some babies seem to know what to do from the start. Others need help and a little time to learn how, like Anne's baby, Alan: *"Alan seemed to have trouble latching on."*

Stroke your baby's cheek gently to encourage her interest in nursing.

Wait for your baby's mouth to open wide.

A good mouthful, with more of the areola from underneath the nipple in the baby's mouth.

Support your breast without compressing any milk ducts.

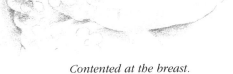

Contented at the breast.

FEEDING FILE

Looking at the baby's position

Although breastfeeding is a natural process, it is also a skill to be learned. Getting the right position at the beginning will help prevent many problems later on.

Beginning with you

First, find a comfortable place to nurse. Sit in a chair or lie on the bed. Make sure that your back is well supported. Sit upright, not leaning back or tipping forward. Don't sit up in bed. It is very hard to sit upright in bed without slipping. Have a drink and perhaps a snack at hand. Many women find that they feel thirsty when the baby begins to nurse.

Support the baby's weight with pillows. There should no strain on your back. The baby should face you, with her head, neck and back in a straight line. Her head should not have to turn to reach the nipple. That would make it hard for her to swallow. She needs to have her nose in line with your nipple, with her body tucked in close to yours. This helps the baby take more of the breast tissue into her mouth from below the nipple. This is where most of the action of the baby's jaw and tongue works to strip milk from the breast.

Latching on

Your baby may already be searching around for the nipple. If not, touch her lips with your nipple or stroke her cheek. Wait for the baby's mouth to open wide so she can take a large mouthful of breast. Her tongue should be down, not on the roof of her mouth. When, and only when, her mouth is wide open, the baby can be moved swiftly towards your breast and allowed to latch on. Be patient. She will get there. She should have her head tilted back, with her chin stretched upwards,

not tucked into her chest. Her body needs to be in line with yours, closely tucked in. She will have more of the areola from underneath the nipple in her mouth than from on top, because it is her tongue and lower jaw that do the work of stripping the milk from the breast. Don't force the whole areola into her mouth. As long as she takes a good mouthful, she'll be fine.

You may not need to hold your breast at all. But if you feel better doing so, then hold your hand palm upwards, with your little finger against your ribcage. Let your breast rest on the flat of your hand. Or, rest the fingers of your hand against your ribcage, with your thumb held away from the breast. With these positions, you won't compress any of the milk ducts. The "scissors" hold, pinching the breast between the index and middle finger, keeps the milk from flowing through the ducts under the fingers and could lead to a blockage.

Sucking

The baby will begin to suck strongly. At first, her sucking pattern will be regular, with even, short sucks. Once the milk has let down, the pattern changes to a few rapid sucks, a pause, then slower, longer, drawing sucks and a swallow. As the feeding progresses, she will suck, draw, swallow and pause. Pauses are a natural part of nursing. They do not usually mean she has had enough. When she has had enough, she will release the suction and push the breast out of her mouth.

FEEDING FILE (continued)

Sucking

If the baby is latched on well, the sensation may be strong. You should not feel any pain. If it is painful, the baby's suction can be gently released by inserting a little finger into the side of her mouth. Although it is tempting to keep nursing in case the pain goes away, this is a mistake. It is much better to start again. Wait for the baby to offer a wide-open mouth.

A good latch

If the baby seems calm and content and you are comfortable, he is probably latched on well. Other signs to look for include the muscles of his face working. You may even see his ears "wiggle," but this may not be obvious. You may hear the sound of milk being swallowed or feel milk being let down. Some mothers, but not all—six out of 10—feel a warm, tingling sensation as this happens. Most of all, your baby will be calm and content and enjoying his feeding.

Both breasts

It is very important to let the baby decide for himself how long he wants to stay on the first breast. Once he has enough and has let go of the nipple, move him over to the other breast. Burping is not essential, but some mothers like to do it. Go through the steps to get the position right once again on this side. Take time to get it right. Once the baby is latched on well, let him nurse for as long as he wants at this breast. He may only want to "finish up" at this breast. You might want to start with this breast first the next time he wants to nurse, to keep from getting lopsided.

Colostrum to mature milk

Once your colostrum begins to change to mature milk, your breasts may feel sore, hot and hard. This is because of increased blood flow to the breasts, combined with tissue swelling as the milk "comes in." If you have been nursing your baby whenever he wants, this uncomfortable fullness should last for only a short time. Often, the breasts will feel better in 24 to 48 hours.

After the initial fullness has passed, your breasts may continue to feel full before your baby has a feeding. They will feel softer and less full after your baby has nursed. After a few weeks, your breasts settle into providing the milk required at each feeding, so you may not notice much difference, if any, before and after nursing. This does not mean that you have less milk. It just means that your supply is now well established. Breastfeeding will be a part of your life for as long as you both want it to be.

CHECKLIST

The baby's position— Have I got it right?

You should see:
- A relaxed, happy baby
- Chest to chest—tucked in close to you
- Chin to breast—head back and chin forward
- A wide-open mouth, with bottom lip turned out, not sucked in
- More breast in baby's mouth below nipple than above
- Face and jaw muscles working. You may see "wiggling" ears.

You should not see:
- Pinched, "prissy" lips
- Baby's cheeks being sucked in.

You will hear:
- Sounds of milk being swallowed. A change from quick, small sucks to deeper, satisfied gulps as the milk is released from the breast.

You should not hear:
- Clicking noises
- Lip smacking

You may feel:
- Your let-down reflex working— a tingling, warm feeling
- Feelings of pleasure and enjoyment

You should not feel:
- Pain that continues throughout the feeding

"He would cry to be fed but then would become frantic quickly. Even the touch of a nipple against his face did not get him to suck and settle down. While he cried, his mouth would be open wide but it wouldn't close over the nipple. But if I tried to nurse him before he started screaming, he wouldn't open his mouth wide enough to latch on right."

Judy found it easier: *"From the start, he would nipple-search with a mouth that looked like a small underpass. I'm sure that this helped a lot. There was no 'leaping' on my part to get the nipple in while his mouth was open. He'd just wait for it and then clamp down."*

Let Down

If your baby is well-positioned at the breast, he will drink the sweet foremilk first. As the hormone oxytocin flows into the bloodstream, it makes the milk-producing cells contract. They squeeze the hindmilk into the ducts, where it is ready for the baby. The squeezing of milk into the ducts is called the *let-down reflex*.

Some women feel the let down as a pleasant sensation. Others report it as a tingling feeling. A few may feel it is painful, particularly in the early days. About 60% of women do not feel anything at all in their breasts when their hindmilk is released, but the baby thrives and receives plenty of breast milk. If you do feel a sensation, you may find it comforting. If you can feel it flowing, there must be milk in your breasts. These are a few of the feelings some mothers report:

"As for the let-down reflex—it can be quite sharp. But I didn't feel it was painful. Pleasurable? Sometimes, yes—especially if I was nursing in a relaxed way and in harmony with the baby. It adds to the feeling of nurturing, of giving life and nourishment."

"I think the pain was caused by the let-down reflex working. It lasted for six weeks."

"I expected to feel the let-down reflex and some kind of sensation when the baby nursed. But I didn't feel anything."

"The feeling when my milk 'lets down' is not like anything I've ever felt before. My nipples and breasts tingle and feel warm. And I feel very relaxed and in love with my baby."

BACKGROUND NOTES

After-pains

Your uterus continues to contract at intervals after labor is over. Contractions last for a few days. Breastfeeding is a time when you might notice these "after-pains." The hormone that releases your milk, oxytocin, contracts your uterus at the same time. This is your body's way of helping you get back into shape quickly.

If this is your first baby, you may not notice these contractions. With second or subsequent babies, you will probably feel them. They may feel like strong menstrual cramps. Once your uterus has regained its pre-pregnancy size, the contractions cease. The pains will go away.

It may help to remember that you will be back in shape sooner than a mother who does not breastfeed!

Unrestricted Feedings

It used to be that mothers were advised to breastfeed at fixed intervals, such as every four hours, and for certain lengths of time, such as 10 minutes per side. This schedule was thought to protect the baby from digestive problems from overfeeding and to prevent sore nipples. But, although some babies may only want to nurse every four hours, most will want to nurse more often. Many will want to nurse much more often. The time between feedings varies from baby to baby and even from hour to hour for the same baby. The only constant is that there is no constant.[33]

Babies who determine the timing of their feedings themselves gain weight more quickly. They are much more likely to breastfeed for a longer time than those whose feedings are restricted or timed in some way.[33]

Research shows that limiting sucking time does not prevent sore nipples. Sore nipples are normally caused by a poor position of the baby at the breast, not by the sucking itself. Limiting the baby's time at the breast can cause more problems.[34] The baby needs enough time at the breast to get a balanced meal of both foremilk and hindmilk. The feeding starts with lower-calorie foremilk. As the volume decreases, foremilk is followed by higher-calorie hindmilk. Most healthcare providers have changed their practice to be in line with this research. It has become rare to find a doctor or nurse advising a mother to limit her baby's nursing to protect her nipples. But some mothers may still hear this advice:

"I was encouraged to nurse on demand, which meant every two hours and sometimes hourly. I found this really tiring. This was my first baby and I had a very difficult and long birth."

"I was warned by an experienced midwife not to let him suck for longer than a few minutes on each side. She told me this could lead to sore nipples. So I would pry him off after the prescribed time."

In some hospitals, even though the baby's sucking time at the breast is not restricted, you may find rules about the time allotted between feedings. You may be asked to wake your baby after a certain time if she is not awake for a feeding. There is rarely any need to wake a healthy full-term baby.

Most mothers find that, even if they try to "obey the rules," their baby will not nurse until she is hungry, as Colette discovered: *"After the first little feeding right after birth, Graham slept for six hours. The hospital nurse, who was pretty old-fashioned anyway, said he shouldn't go any longer than that without a feeding. She insisted on waking him up by putting water on his face. She said he would dehydrate if he didn't get some fluids. I felt at the time that this had to be wrong. He was a perfectly healthy baby. But needless to say, I gave in to her 'superior knowledge' and let her wake him up. He didn't take more than a few sucks. I learned later that women having second or subsequent babies in the same hospital were not treated this way. They and their babies were allowed to sleep until the baby woke up on his own."*

Sleepy Babies

Research studies on normal babies' feeding habits show that feedings are often infrequent for the first few days. Some reluctance to nurse at the start may be perfectly normal. A baby may refuse to suck because of pain-relief medication the mother took during labor. Most pain relief medications pass quickly through the placenta to the baby. Their effects can be long-lasting.

Some babies who are sleepy after birth are developing jaundice. A jaundiced baby's skin looks yellow. He may not care to nurse for very long. And he may fall asleep after only a few sucks. Jaundice that develops around the second to fourth day is so common that it is known as *physiologic jaundice*. One of the best ways to reduce this type of jaundice is frequent nursing. But because jaundice can make a baby sleepy, this may not be easy. Extra fluids, such as water, may be offered in a mistaken attempt to "flush out" the jaundice. However, water has no effect on jaundice. It will only fill the baby's stomach so he does not want to breastfeed.

Janice's labor was induced when she was 38 weeks pregnant after having a prenatal hemorrhage (sudden bleeding) at 36 weeks. Her baby was fine except for being a little jaundiced and very sleepy: *"The nurses wanted me to give him extra fluids, mainly water, because of the jaundice. But I declined. Instead, we would wake him to nurse as often as possible because he was so sleepy. He did well once my milk supply was established and we were settled at home."*

Sometimes, if the levels of jaundice are high, the baby will be treated with *phototherapy*. This involves putting the baby under bright white lights, usually with his eyes covered. Phototherapy reduces the jaundice. But it can also make the baby cranky.

One form of jaundice starts toward the end of the first week of life. It may last for several weeks. It is often called *breast-milk jaundice* and seems to be found in breastfed babies with no other obvious symptoms except yellowness. There are several theories about what causes this, but no one knows which is correct.

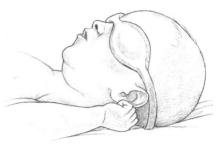

BACKGROUND NOTES

Jaundice

In the first week of life, many babies become jaundiced. Most of these babies are not ill. Only one baby in a thousand[35] will have something wrong: a problem with the liver or a blood-group incompatibility. Most jaundiced babies have "physiologic" jaundice, caused by a natural process as the baby adapts to life outside the womb. This form of jaundice is harmless. It rarely requires treatment, and you don't need to check into it to determine the cause.

During pregnancy, the fetus does not breathe for himself. He needs extra red blood cells to get all the oxygen he needs. After birth, he does breathe for himself. So those extra red blood cells are no longer needed. When red blood cells are broken down by the liver, they produce *bilirubin*. Bilirubin makes the baby's skin yellow.

Because the baby's liver is immature, it cannot get rid of the bilirubin very well. It takes 3 to 5 days for the liver to mature. In the meantime, bilirubin can collect and cause jaundice. Jaundice can be worsened by bruising at birth. Drugs given to the mother in pregnancy or during labor (oxytocin or epidural anesthesia) can also worsen jaundice.

"Early" jaundice, which begins in the first 24 hours of life, is a sign there may be a more serious cause for concern. Medical treatment may be needed. Jaundice may also be more serious in a baby born prematurely.

Sometimes jaundice starts later, towards the end of the first week of life. If there are no other symptoms, there is usually no cause for concern. This type of jaundice is sometimes called "breast-milk" jaundice. In an otherwise healthy, thriving breastfed baby there is no reason to take the baby off the breast to "diagnose" the condition, as healthcare providers sometimes suggest.[35]

Is treatment necessary?

The best treatment for jaundice in a breastfed baby is to nurse the baby more often—about 12 times a day. Extra fluids, other than breast milk, are not needed and may be harmful.[36] A baby with jaundice tends to be sleepy. He may need to be stimulated, perhaps by changing his diaper. He may not want to nurse for very long for a few days. Still, it is important to offer the breast frequently until the jaundice passes, because your colostrum helps your baby pass the sticky meconium in his bowels. The longer the meconium stays in the bowels, the greater the chance of jaundice.

Bilirubin is fat-soluble, so food (especially hindmilk) helps it to pass more quickly. Water can't do this. If your baby is not taking much milk, try expressing to maintain your milk supply until the baby is ready for a longer feeding. Expressed milk can also be fed to the baby from a cup or spoon.

If your baby needs phototherapy, it is still important to breastfeed frequently. Make sure that phototherapy really is needed. Babies have to be placed naked under white lights. The light contains a blue spectrum, which changes bilirubin into another harmless substance. Their eyes are often covered for protection. Babies may become fussy and cranky under the lights. They may develop diarrhea. Babies who undergo phototherapy will lose more water through their skin and will need to drink more. For a breastfed baby, this extra fluid can always be breast milk.

It used to be suggested that breastfeeding be stopped for 24 hours to confirm the diagnosis. Now we know there is no reason for doing this. Stopping breastfeeding distresses mother and baby and does not achieve very much. It's true the levels of jaundice may fall a little more quickly if you stop nursing. But they will also disappear without *any* treatment, as Ellen's baby George's did: *"The beginning with George was easy. He took to breastfeeding—no problem! I was relaxed and confident. But he was still jaundiced at four weeks. We went to the hospital for blood tests. The verdict was breast-milk jaundice. What a shame so much blood had to be sucked out of him and so many tests taken, just to satisfy the doctors! At least nobody suggested I should stop nursing him. By six weeks it had passed, and he lost his 'tan.'"*

Inverted Nipples

About 2% of women have inverted nipples. If your nipples look like craters and do not stand out when you are cold or during love-making, or turn further inwards, they are considered "inverted". Many mothers with inverted nipples are discouraged from trying to breastfeed. But let's remember that the baby is breastfeeding, not nipple feeding! With the correct position, your baby should be able to take in a good mouthful of breast. Erect nipples are useful but not essential for breastfeeding.

Given good support and help with the baby's position, mothers with flat or inverted nipples can breastfeed as well as anyone else, as Teresa found out: *"During my first pregnancy I felt that, for me, breastfeeding was a very important part of becoming a mother. I was strongly motivated to succeed. But I was warned by doctors and nurses that there could be real problems because my nipples have always been fully inverted. On a cold day I look like I have Lifesavers® candy under my sweater—complete with holes! They could not be coaxed out at all. All my massaging and wearing breast shields had no effect. I felt it might not be possible, but I'd do my best.*

"Tim arrived two weeks early. He didn't latch on easily or seem to have a very strong suck. It wasn't easy. The hospital nurses began to doubt I had any colostrum. But before the birth, slight pressure had expressed a little fluid, so I felt this wasn't the case. Well-meaning nurses tried to squeeze my apparently nipple-less areolas into Tim's mouth. This left us both feeling tired and frustrated. It did nothing for my

dignity, confidence or privacy. I tried using nipple shields, which helped a little. I was reassured by the sight of milk in the shield at the end of a feeding.

"I was relieved to get home and contact my local La Leche League leader. Despite pressure from doctors and nurses to give Tim bottles of formula, I kept these to an absolute minimum. I spent my time cuddling and nursing as much as possible.

"There were times when I was very sore, tired and frustrated. I needed the support and encouragement of my husband, La Leche League counselor and friends. Our efforts were rewarded when my nipples began to feel better. I realized that Tim didn't need large nipples to 'suck.' He could milk the breast quite well without them.

"My nipples did begin to appear during feedings—seeing light of day for the first time in my 41 years! I was very sore and a little frightened by it. It was often very uncomfortable, sometimes painful, and looked strange and unfamiliar. My nipples changed a lot. Little skin tags hardened and later fell off. Then a softer, natural-looking nipple emerged for feedings. They were never erect or ready for Tim, who had to draw them out at the start of each feeding. If anyone with inverted nipples considers NOT trying to breastfeed her baby, I would strongly advise her to think again. Like me, she may find it difficult. But the pain and heartache will soon give way to real comfort and pleasure. It's something I wouldn't have missed for the world."

Fullness When the Milk Comes In

If you feed your baby frequently from birth, you may not become over-full as the milk comes in. If your breasts do become very full and hard (*engorged*) when the milk comes in, you may have trouble latching on the baby and need extra help.

When Susan's milk came in, her baby had just gone to sleep after being awake and nursing for several hours. She used the electric pump in the hospital to remove just enough milk to relieve the pressure in her breasts: *"After that, if my breasts were too hard and the nipple and areola too taut for the baby to latch on to, I put warm washcloths on my breasts. That got the milk flowing. The nipple got softer and she could latch on."*

Elaine had such a fierce let down that milk sprayed out everywhere at first: *"It made my breasts softer and easier to latch David on to. But my nipples were so sore it was agony. He only nursed from one side and fell asleep. I changed his diaper and tried to get him to take the other side. But he didn't want it and fell asleep again. I was left with one breast that felt like a lump of concrete. I called my mom and she suggested a warm bath and using warm washcloths to soothe it. That night my milk came in and I became completely engorged. I awoke exhausted from a night of trying to latch on a screaming baby.*

"I called my mom again and she came over. She suggested that I nurse from the most painful side, and helped me latch David on. He nursed for 30 minutes solid, then fell asleep. I was still uncomfortable on the other side, with no prospect of a feeding for a couple of hours. So Mom suggested that I try (unsuccessfully) to gently hand-express a little milk, to ease the discomfort. I ended up having another warm bath, putting lots of warm washcloths on my breasts."

Anna tried out a tip she had heard about: *"In the hospital I became painfully engorged on the third day. I found the value in half-frozen Savoy cabbage leaves—bliss when worn inside a good supportive bra and changed frequently. Not sure about the smell, but at the time I didn't care."*

In most cases, this painful fullness passes within 24 to 48 hours. It can be eased by getting the milk to flow.

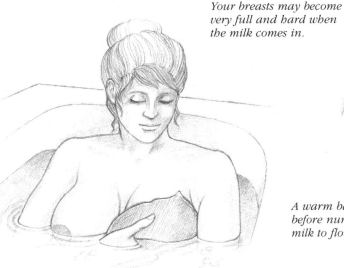

Your breasts may become very full and hard when the milk comes in.

A warm bath, especially before nursing, helps the milk to flow.

FEEDING FILE

Coping with fullness when the milk "comes in"

Many mothers find their breasts change around the third or fourth day after the birth, from being soft to being firm and full. The milk is changing from colostrum to mature milk. The blood and lymph supply to your breasts has increased. There is fluid (*edema*) in your breast tissues. Your breasts may feel hot and hard. You may feel some pain. This is often called *engorgement*. This condition will only last for 24 to 48 hours. If you feed your baby very frequently from birth, you may not become engorged at all.

How to cope

- Most important, feed your baby often, for as long as she wants.

- If you are very full, you may need to soften the nipple to help your baby latch on. If your nipples are not standing out as much as they were, your baby may have some trouble taking in enough breast tissue. It can be easy to get sore nipples if she is not taking a good mouthful.

- Massage your nipples gently.

- Do be gentle with anything you do. Your breast tissue can bruise easily at this sensitive time.

- Alternate warmth and cold. Warm washcloths, or a warm shower, especially before nursing, helps milk flow. An ice-pack wrapped in a dishtowel, or even a packet of frozen peas, helps soothe the breasts, especially after nursing.

- Some mothers find that cabbage leaves chilled in the refrigerator are soothing when slipped around the breast inside their bra. Leave them in place for half an hour or so, until they reach body temperature.

- Try using a breast pump, hand or electric, just before nursing. If you become uncomfortable before your baby wants to nurse again, express a little milk until you feel better.

- Make sure that your bra is not too tight. Any constriction could lead to bruising and blocked ducts or *mastitis* (an inflamed or swollen breast).

- Ask your healthcare provider for a suitable painkiller, such as acetaminophen [as in Tylenol®] or ibuprofen [as in Advil®] if you need one. They will not harm your baby.

BREASTMILK PRODUCTION FROM BIRTH

Age of the baby	Volume per day		Volume per feeding	
	Range	Average	On Average	Refs.
Day 1 (0-24 hours)	7-123mls	37mls	7mls	1,3,5
Day 2 (24-48 hours)	44-335mls	84mls	14mls	3
Day 3 (48-72 hours)	98-775mls	408mls	38mls	1,2,3
Day 4 (72-96 hours)	375-876mls	625mls	58mls	1,3
Day 5 (95-120 hours)	452-876mls	700mls	70mls	1,3
3 months	609-837mls	750mls		4
6 months		800ml		

References

1. Saint, L., Smith, M. and Harmann, P. 1984: The yield and nutrient content of colostrum and milk from giving birth to one month postpartum. *British Journal of Nutrition,* vol. 52: pp. 87-95.

2. Neville, M. et al. 1988: Studies in human lactation: milk volumes in lactating women during the onset of lactation and full lactation. *American Society for Clinical Nutrition,* vol. 48: pp. 1375-1386.

3. Houston, M. J., Howie, P. and McNeilly, A. S. 1983: Factors affecting the duration of breastfeeding: 1. Measurement of breast milk intake in the first week of life. *Early Human Development,* vol. 8: pp. 49-54.

4. Butte, N., Garza, C., O'Brian Smith, E. and Nichols, B. L. 1984: Human milk intake and growth in exclusively breastfed infants. *Journal of Pediatrics,* vol. 104: pp. 187-195.

5. Roderuck, C., Williams, H. H. and Macy, J. G. 1946: *Journal of Nutrition,* vol. 32: pp. 267-283.

REAL-LIFE BREASTFEEDING: THE FIRST TWO WEEKS

At the start of your baby's life, it can seem as if your baby is totally unpredictable. You never know when she is going to sleep and for how long, stay awake or want another feeding. If you relax and follow your baby's lead, you will find that after a while she will begin to develop some kind of pattern. Rayanne recorded the first 14 days of her third baby Connie's life. She noted when Connie nursed, when she slept and when she was awake without wanting to nurse. We have reproduced an example of those records below.

DAY 2

Slept from midnight to 5 am. Nursed on and off from 5 am to 8:30 am. Slept to 12:30 pm. Nursed from 12:30 pm to 1:30 pm. Slept from 1:30 pm to 3:30 pm. Nursed and changed at 4 pm. Nursed again at 5 pm and about 6 pm. Fussy, nursed again at 7 pm and finally slept until 11 pm. Nursed on and off throughout the night while I slept.

DAY 4

Nursed until about 12:30 am. Slept for about 10 minutes, then was awake and nursing on and off most of the night in my bed. Nursed at 6 am and slept until 10 am. Nursed and was awake for a while. Bathed and nursed again to settle back to sleep at about 12:30 pm. Slept until 3:45 pm. Nursed for about half an hour. Awake, being cuddled, etc. Nursed again at 5:30 pm for a short while, slept until 9 pm. Awake, nursed again at 10:15 pm. Changed, nursed again. Slept from 11:15 pm to 2 am.

Day 7

Nursed at 2:15 am. Slept until 5:45 am, nursed. Slept until 9 am, nursed until 10 am. Awake—cuddles and changing etc. Back to sleep at 11:30 am. Slept until 1 pm. Nursed and changed. First excursion out shopping. Slept all afternoon in the stroller. Nursed at 4:30 pm. Changed, nursed again at 5:30 pm. Changed, nursed again at 6:30 pm. Back to sleep at 7 pm until 10:30 pm. Nursed until 11:30 pm, awake.

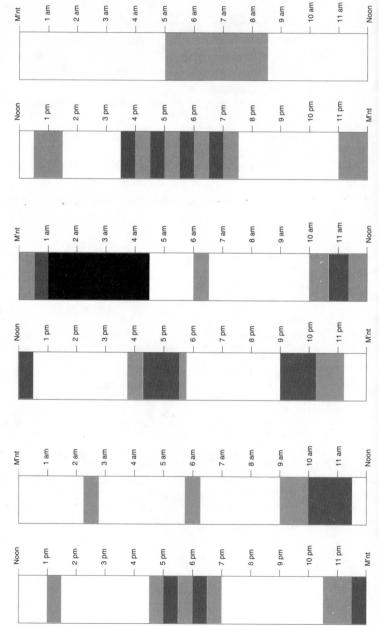

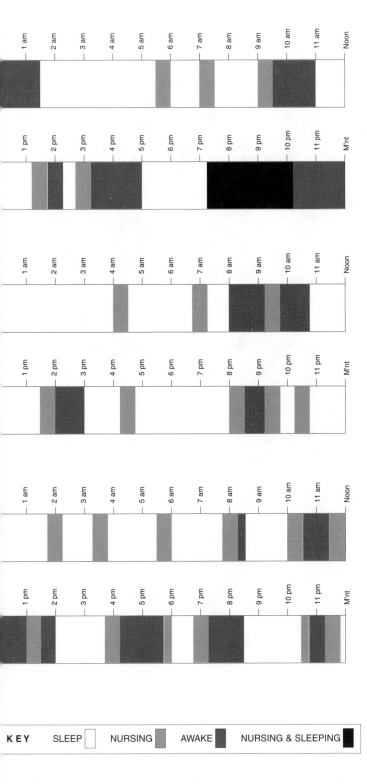

DAY 10

Slept from 1:30 am until 5:30 am, nursed. Slept. Nursed again at 7 am. Slept again until 9 am. Nursed, awake. Bathed. Settled to sleep at 11 am. Slept until 1:10 pm. Nursed on and off for about an hour. Nursed again, awake, then settled to sleep at 5 pm. Slept until 7:10 pm. Nursed, slept until 10:15 pm. Nursed, awake until 12:15 am.

DAY 12

Woke for a feeding at 4 am. Nursed, slept, nursed again at 6:45 am. Slept. Woke at 8 am, dozed and cried in the car. Nursed at 9:10 am, changed, awake. Settled to sleep at 10:45 am. Woke at 1:30 pm, nursed, changed, awake. Dozed in car. Nursed at 4:10 pm. Slept until 8 pm. Nursed, awake, nursed again at 9:15 pm. Slept. Changed, nursed, slept at 10:45 pm .

DAY 14

Slept until 1:45 am. Nursed, slept. Nursed again at 3:15 am and 5:35 am. Slept and nursed again at 7:45 am. Changed, slept from 8:30 am until 10 am. Nursed, awake, nursed again. Awake. Nursed at 1 pm. Awake. Slept from 2 pm until 3:45 pm. Nursed, awake, nursed again at 5:45 pm. Slept from 6 pm to 6:40. Nursed, fell asleep at 8:30 pm until 10:30 pm. Nursed on and off until 11:45 pm. Settled to sleep.

KEY   SLEEP   NURSING   AWAKE   NURSING & SLEEPING

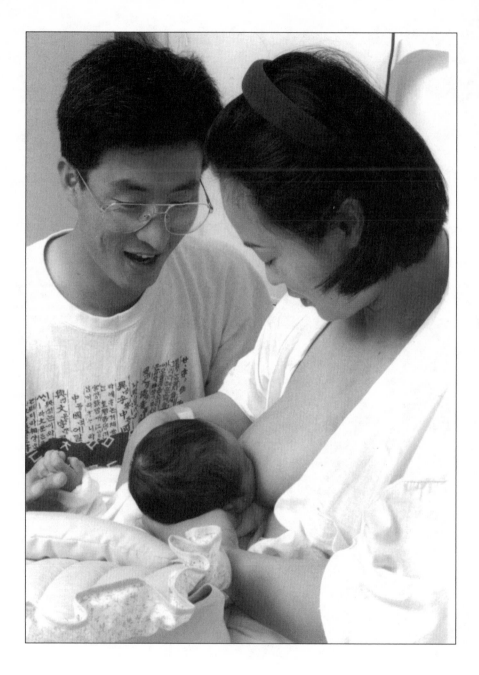

CHAPTER 3

Helping Hands

Nurses and midwives in hospitals and birthing centers are beginning to realize they play a crucial role in helping a mother start to breastfeed successfully. Hospitals perhaps have not always been the best place for learning to breastfeed.[37] In the United States and Canada, UNICEF's Baby Friendly Hospital Initiative (BFHI) is working to raise the awareness of good practice in hospitals. Policies to protect and support breastfeeding, which everyone knows about, are beginning to be practiced in maternity units throughout Canada and the United States. New mothers are profoundly influenced by the attitudes and practices of staff in hospitals and birthing centers.[38] If the hospital staff believe in and support breastfeeding, the mothers they meet will succeed.

A Good Start

Various things can help you and your baby get off to a good start with breastfeeding. One of the most important is positive support and encouragement from health providers, friends and family. At first, many mothers lack confidence in their ability to breastfeed successfully. They are vulnerable to critical comments. This is not meant to suggest that if you don't receive positive support, you are doomed to failure with breastfeeding. But starting to breastfeed is much easier if, like Cindy, you feel that those around you want you to succeed and believe you can do so: *"There was a fantastic breastfeeding nurse at the hospital at the time (who has now retired). She gave me the best support in the first few days. She was so calm and positive. She gave me confidence in myself and my ability to nurse my baby. She got me through a very bad case of 'four-day blues.'"*

On the second day, Emily's baby, Hugh, seemed fussy. He was her second baby and she was—at least to start with—fairly confident. But she found herself wondering what she was doing wrong. Instead, she could have thought of him as a newborn baby who might take a while to adjust to the world outside: *"Was I not giving him enough? Too much? He was nursing a lot more often than the two bottle-fed babies next to us. A nurse suggested I try some water to help him burp. He wasn't very interested and it didn't seem to help. Another nurse advised a bottle of formula. Maybe the colostrum wasn't filling enough and he was hungry. I knew that the colostrum was highly nutritious and should be all that he needed. But after he'd cried on and off all evening, I was beginning to have doubts about the whole thing.*

"The staff and other mothers were nice about the crying. But everyone suggested I change the way I was feeding Hugh so he'd stop crying. That was hard on me. I really needed someone to say 'You're doing fine. Don't worry. He'll settle down soon.' We left the hospital on the fourth day. Hugh was weighed before we went. He'd regained his birthweight, plus a little, which was a big boost to my confidence."

Clear and Consistent Information

A second key factor for a successful start to breastfeeding is good, clear, consistent advice and information, based on an agreed policy. Some hospitals and birthing centers already have such policies. Others are developing them. Once a policy exists, a lot of effort and staff training may be needed to ensure it is put into practice. It's easy to see how a mother could receive conflicting advice if such a policy doesn't exist. Getting a lot of contradictory information can be extremely confusing when you are trying to learn something new.

Before offering advice, a nurse might help by asking what advice you have been offered already—and by whom. Or you might tell your healthcare practitioner what you were already told and how you felt about it. If a hospital has a clear policy on breastfeeding, which they tell you about, you may not hear the kinds of confusing messages that Stacy received: *"I wasn't helped by the different advice I got from every nurse I met—often a different nurse at each feeding. They were all kind and helpful. But each one had a different opinion about how to deal with Daniel's refusal to nurse. There was no overall plan to follow."*

When Joy moved from the teaching hospital to the local community hospital, things improved a lot: *"The staff was a little out-of-date on breastfeeding. They still pushed feedings every four hours. But luckily Maggie wanted to nurse about every four hours at that stage. The wonderful thing was that they all said the same thing. And they wanted me to succeed with breastfeeding."*

Elaine received conflicting advice on the very first day: *"After David was born, he was very alert and looked at me very intently. When I tried to put him to my breast about 30 minutes after he was born, one of the aides cleaning up the delivery room said: 'Oh, you don't want to do that yet. Give him a chance! He probably just wants to cuddle.' I felt totally embarrassed and quickly covered myself up. I felt stupid and wanted someone to help me desperately, but I didn't dare ask. I just sat there with tears pouring down my cheeks hugging David to me. About two hours later, a nurse-midwife asked me if I had nursed David. She was surprised when I said that I hadn't, and told me that I could have done it right away. She helped me latch David on. It felt strange at first, to have a slight tugging feeling at my breast. But I relaxed and soon realized I was beaming. I felt so proud of myself and my baby! It seemed the most natural thing in the world. I forgot everything and everyone else in those first exciting minutes."*

Supplementary Liquids

Breastfed babies do not need any other fluids besides breast milk. Sometimes, however, extra fluids are suggested for several reasons. These include thirst (and hot weather); jaundice; and hunger, either because the milk has not yet "come in," or because breastfeeding seems to have "failed." These are not valid reasons for giving formula, water or any other fluid. A healthy baby does not need large volumes of fluid before it becomes available from the breast.[33] Giving a breastfed baby anything other than breast milk in the first few days could confuse her. In some cases, it may lead to the end of breastfeeding. For example, in the 1990 Infant Feeding Survey,[1] 32% of mothers whose breastfed babies also received bottles of formula in the hospital stopped breastfeeding in the first two weeks, compared with 9% of mothers whose babies did not receive formula.

FEEDING FILE

Coping with Conflicting Advice

As a new mother, you may feel unsure about how to handle, comfort and feed your baby. You may want to ask other people what to do about a particular question. And lots of people may want to "tell" you what to do, whether you ask or not. They want to give you advice.

Typical advice-giving statements begin with:

- "'If I were you, I'd . . .'"
- "When my baby was two days old, I . . ."
- "If you don't do X, then Y will happen."
- "Stop breastfeeding now because . . ."
- "It's because you are breastfeeding that . . ."
- "You really ought to . . ."
- "You must . . ."

Each one of these statements may end with a different suggestion. A lot of conflicting advice may leave a new mother feeling confused.

Tips for coping with conflicting advice

- Have an idea of how you would like to feed your baby.
- Try to choose one person whom you trust, and listen to her.
- Remember that no one can "make" you do what you do not want to do for yourself or your baby.
- You are the baby's mother. It is highly likely that you know your baby better than anyone else.

- You do not need to try all the advice you are offered. Try only what seems right for you and your baby. Remember some advice for later and throw out the rest.
- Ask why what is being suggested might work.
- If you are uneasy with advice, ask if there is research to support the suggestion.
- If you do not feel able to listen to any more advice from outsiders, ask your partner, friend or relative—whoever is closest to you at the time—to shield you from it.
- If you are assertive and sound confident about what you are doing, most compulsive advice-givers retreat.
- It's possible that a simple "recipe" such as feeding your baby when he is hungry, comforting him when he cries and helping him to sleep when he is tired, could work for you.
- Contact a lactation consultant or La Leche League leader. She will listen and support you in your decision-making. If she does not know the answer right away, she will be able to find out and give you information based on current research.

Elaine feels she was pressured into giving her baby a bottle: *"At least one nurse suggested that David was hungry because my milk hadn't come in. Since I needed my sleep, why didn't I just let them give him a little formula to tide him over? I was emotional and vulnerable. I began to feel that I was depriving David of something and exhausting myself in the process. So I gave in during the night. A very smug nurse told me that he had guzzled down a bottle and was now sound asleep. Did I feel inadequate! Luckily that only happened once and then 'the milk came in'—as if what comes before is useless!"*

Carol's experience was similar: *"The second night my nice nurse was off, replaced by a bossy one who scared me. And of course my baby woke for the night. The first part of the night we fought. She wanted to take him to the nursery and give him a bottle of formula. She watched me nurse, which made me feel awkward and embarrassed. She said my baby was not getting enough milk, was hungry and that I had to get some rest and stop disturbing the people around me. Finally she stormed over and wheeled my baby away for the rest of the night. I do not know if she gave him a bottle or not."*

Colostrum, the first milk your baby receives from the breast, may come in small amounts but it is highly nutritious and satisfying. It also contains protection from infection for the baby. A baby's stomach at birth is tiny—only about $1\frac{1}{2}$ inches long (about the size of a walnut). It does not take a lot of milk to fill it. Nor is a baby born starving. She has been fully nourished by the placenta, in most cases.

If a baby's hunger and thirst are satisfied by other fluids, she will nurse less at the breast. Regular nursing at the breast, and removal of milk, is essential to help establish a good supply of breast milk. Your confidence in your ability to breastfeed may be undermined if you are led to believe that your milk does not satisfy your baby's needs. In addition, the baby may find it harder to learn to nurse at the breast if she is also learning to drink from a bottle.

In the hospital, if breastfeeding seems difficult, some women may be tempted to give their babies the ready-made "solution" of formula milk, as Sandra was: *"But Helen was clearly hungry. People kept asking me if my milk had come in and telling me that sometimes it didn't come in until the fifth day after a C-section. I was persuaded to give her some*

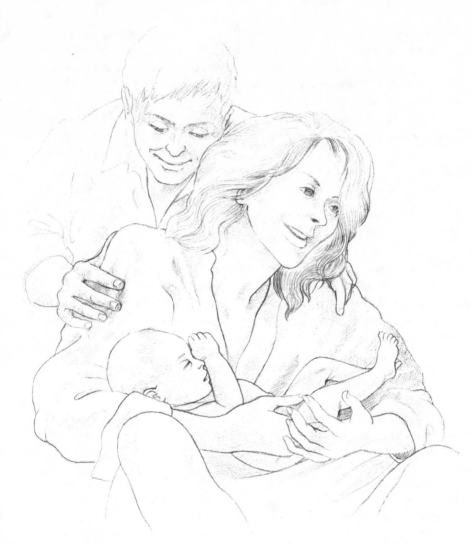

expressed breast milk from the neonatal intensive care unit. After two or three days, I felt so guilty about using this that I gave her a bottle of formula. I wanted to breastfeed so much, to get something right after the perceived failure of my emergency Cesarean. I knew also that giving my baby bottles might stop her from sucking properly at the breast, because a bottle is so much easier to get milk from. And I knew that worry itself could stop the let-down reflex. I was getting more and more depressed. I think I spent most of the time in tears."

Low Blood Sugar

Some hospitals are concerned if a baby is not fed at regular intervals, especially if there is a long interval between the birth and the baby's first feeding. This seems to worry nurses more if the baby is heavy at birth. One concern is that the baby may become "jittery" or hypoglycemic (get low blood sugar). This is often the time when pressure may be brought to bear on you to give your baby a bottle of formula milk, as these three women remember with regret:

"Then the nurse said that because Alison was a very large baby (9 lb. 4 oz.), her blood-sugar levels would be low and would drop further unless she were given supplementary bottles. I was confused and saddened by this and said I didn't want to bottle-feed. The nurse didn't reply. She looked so serious! I couldn't disobey her instructions."

"On the second night, after 20 hours of poor feedings, Tessa's blood-sugar levels were checked. I was told she needed a bottle and was undernourished. I said I wanted to breastfeed but was told it wasn't working. What was I going to do when I got home? And how did I expect to care for her if I didn't even have bottles as a back-up? What little confidence I had left ebbed away. I felt like a total failure, extremely tired and alone. So I agreed for her to be taken away and fed while I tried to sleep."

"My son weighed in at 5 lb. 14 oz. and I was exhausted. However, he was put to the breast right away because I'd made it clear I was going to breastfeed. I got lots of support (with a lot of conflicting advice). But by all accounts I was doing everything right. On the third day, my son weighed only 5 lb. 5 oz. and was miserable. He started to shake uncontrollably. A blood test showed his blood sugar was low and that supplementary bottle-feeding was essential until he regained his weight."

Some mothers are able to resist strong pressure to give extra fluids. Tests done on the baby, such as a heel-prick to test the baby's blood-sugar levels, can be stressful for you and your baby. It is worth asking if the tests are really needed. If the baby shows no other signs of being ill, no supplement may be needed. The best solution is to offer very frequent breastfeedings, so your baby can take as much as she wants from one breast before swapping to the other. This ensures the baby gets the calorie-rich hindmilk. If this is not possible, supplements may be given from a cup or spoon, to keep the baby from being confused by the different sucking action involved in bottle feeding.

BACKGROUND NOTES

Hypoglycemia

Hypoglycemia means *low blood sugar.* For some babies, this may mean they show signs of running out of "fuel" and may become "jittery" or start to have "fits." There is a small risk of brain damage if a baby is deprived for some time of enough "fuel" to function. However, pediatricians have widely different opinions about when low blood sugar is a problem for a baby.[39] As a result, babies are tested and perhaps treated when there is no real need to do so.

It seems that breastfed babies born at full term may be likely to have low blood sugar in the first few days after birth. But they can make and use other fuel stored in their bodies. If they show no symptoms besides a longer interval between feedings in the first few days, they are not ill. They will nurse more often when they are ready.[39]

Measurement

Blood is often taken from the baby's heel using a sharp needle. A drop of blood is smeared on a test strip to measure blood-sugar levels. This test is designed for adult diabetics and not for babies who may have low blood sugar. For babies, the test is not very accurate. The most accurate way to measure blood-sugar levels is by a laboratory blood test.

Treatment

Babies who are thought to have low blood sugar may be offered extra food, often a bottle of formula or dextrose (sugar water). Supplements like these are not necessary in most cases. Breast milk is always the best food to offer.

Early, frequent breastfeeding may prevent hypoglycemia. If the baby is sleepy or will not nurse, and there is cause for concern, expressed breast milk may be offered from a spoon or cup. Babies who are small for their date, premature, or who are born to mothers with diabetes, are more likely to need help. But even these babies may be given expressed breast milk rather than formula.

After 12 hours of Claudette's baby not nursing after birth, the nurse asked her if they could test Emily's blood sugar: *"'If it's OK,' they told me, 'you'll know there's no hurry to feed her.' The test seemed to offer the reassurance I needed, so I consented. Her blood sugar was low, but OK. But Emily still would not nurse for more than a second. She had taken to licking colostrum off my nipples, rather than actually nursing. This seemed to be enough to keep her going. Every two hours, the nurses stuck a needle into Emily to see if her blood sugar was still dropping. I was given a chart and told that Emily had to nurse for at least 20 minutes every four hours if she was going to be all right.*

"As the hours ticked by, I became more and more worried. And the nurses became more and more anxious as I tried to get her to nurse.

They started to mention bottles and hinted that Emily might be ill if she didn't nurse soon. After 24 hours, I was told that Emily's blood sugar was dropping and that I should give her a bottle. 'Just one bottle won't do any harm,' they told me. I said that it could, but the patronizing looks I got in return suggested the nurses didn't believe me. By the way, other women on the ward were having similar problems and they did give their babies bottles. Of six women, I was the only one to go home breastfeeding my baby."

Night Feedings

Breastfeeding during the night is particularly valuable. These feedings seem to stimulate the production of *prolactin,* the hormone involved in making breast milk, much more than feedings during the day.[40] These days, babies often sleep beside their mothers at night, rather than in a nursery, making night feedings easier. Night feedings help to keep your breasts from becoming too full. You can spend time learning to latch your baby onto your breast before the milk comes in. After the milk comes in, your breasts are firm and round, and less easy for the baby to manage for a while. Babies need feeding at night for some weeks. The amount of milk they need will be produced more quickly if night feeding is begun the very first night.

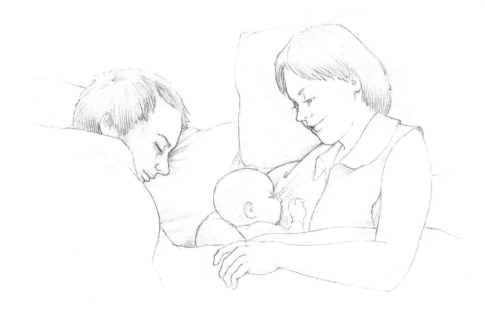

The latest Infant Feeding Survey[1] found that by 1990, 63% of mothers had their babies with them all the time in the hospital, compared with 17% in 1980. This is more likely to encourage mothers to nurse their babies themselves at night, instead of relying on staff to give bottles of formula. Hospital staff may offer to take the baby to the nursery on the first night, so you can rest after the birth. However, most mothers have already found that, by the time they give birth, a "good night's sleep" is a fond memory. At least when you are breastfeeding, you can latch the baby on to your breast and doze while your baby nurses. You won't be worrying whether your baby needs you. Jennifer tried this and has never looked back: *"At 2 a.m., snuffly noises woke me up. I put on my glasses and put him in bed beside me to nurse. I felt so experienced and relaxed this time, like an old hand. The staff wasn't bossy or pushy but just there to make sure we were OK. Richard and I fell asleep. I woke up again at 6 a.m. to find him looking up into my eyes in the half light. Right then I fell hopelessly in love. We changed sides and nodded off again."*

Help with the Baby's Position

Two of the most common reasons for stopping breastfeeding in the first week are the baby's refusal to suck and painful breasts or nipples. In 1990, 36% of mothers who were surveyed reported having nursing

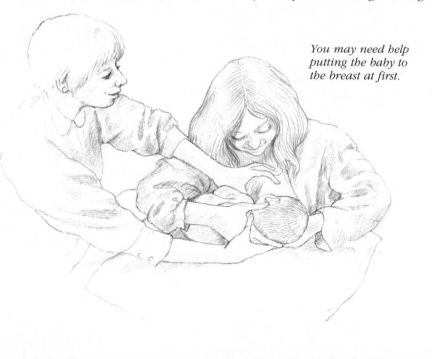

You may need help putting the baby to the breast at first.

problems while in the hospital. The most common problems were trouble in latching the baby on to the breast and sore or cracked nipples. Sunita asked for as much help and advice as she needed: *"I spent most of my time in the hospital with my hand on the buzzer, asking nurses and aides for help in latching Jane on. I had sore nipples for two weeks. I don't know which part of me hurt more, my bottom or my nipples. It was a close thing. I was always convinced that her position was the problem. But no one seemed to really tell me what position Jane should be in. She was just 'latched on' time after time."*

Skilled and experienced help when latching your baby on to the breast in the early days is crucial to successful, pain-free breastfeeding. Jamie felt she needed a lot of help to get Hannah latched on: *"She was a very sleepy baby and needed a lot of encouragement to suck. I thought the nurses and nurse-midwives were wonderful. They stayed with me for as long as it took to get Hannah nursing correctly at nearly every feeding."*

A Relaxing Environment

For some mothers, just being in a hospital makes starting to breastfeed more difficult. Despite the best intentions, hospitals are not often places of peace and quiet. Learning a new and intimate skill such as breastfeeding works best in a quiet, relaxed place. A new family can get to know each other better without strangers walking in on them. Some mothers, however, are glad of 24-hour support and are reluctant to leave the hospital. Some women feel they need an "expert" to guide them in this new role. They may not be quite ready to take on the full responsibility of motherhood and may not feel confident in their ability to cope on their own.

Jean found it hard to breastfeed for the first time in a busy maternity hospital: *"The lady in the next bed was bottle-feeding her second child. There were no curtains around the beds. It was hard to nurse in front of (someone else's) male visitors. Home was 100% better. What peace, to nurse in the comfort of your own bedroom, with comfy pillows and a big bed."*

However, Sarah felt different: *"I didn't look forward to leaving the hospital. How would I manage at home, without all this care and expertise?"*

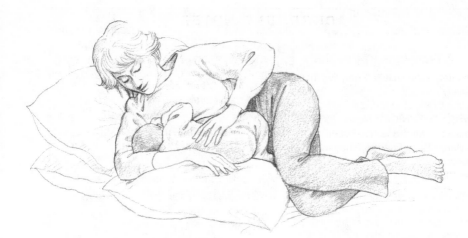

Of course, not all mothers give birth in the hospital. Starting to breast-feed from home may be more peaceful and relaxed, as Ruth relates: *"When my second child was due, I chose to have a home birth. After a three-hour labor, I delivered a 9½-pound baby girl without any inter-vention or drugs. The atmosphere was calm and peaceful. Our sole mid-wife placed the baby in my arms right away, so I could discover the gen-der myself. After the cord had been clamped and cut and the placenta delivered, the midwife left the room to wash up. I placed the baby across my chest, latched her on myself and shared the experience with my hus-band alone. (Our 3-year-old was still sleeping).*

"I felt incredibly close to her. Afterwards we were tucked in together so she could nurse on demand. It was a beautiful, sunny summer's morning and the birds were singing. It couldn't have been more perfect."

What happens in the early days of breastfeeding is very important. During this first week, you and your baby will be learning together and your breastfeeding partnership will be well under way.

BACKGROUND NOTES

A Baby-friendly Hospital?

An international Baby Friendly Hospital Initiative (BFHI) was launched in 1991 by the World Health Organization (WHO) and UNICEF. Nearly 8,000 hospitals worldwide have been declared Baby Friendly. They meet standards set forth in the 10 Steps (see below).

Hospitals and birthing centers in Canada and the United States have just begun the process of becoming certified as "Baby Friendly." Diarrheal and respiratory diseases, the chief killers in the developing world, remain the most common reasons for babies' admission to a hospital in developed countries. Breastfeeding helps protect babies from both kinds of diseases.

The Baby Friendly Hospital Initiative was introduced to encourage hospitals and birthing centers to adopt practices that fully promote and protect exclusive breastfeeding from birth. Baby-friendly hospitals and birthing centers are recognized throughout the world as providers of the highest possible standards of care for breastfeeding mothers and their babies. The primary aim of the Initiative is to return breastfeeding to its rightful place as the most accepted and usual way for a mother to nourish her baby.

The BFHI encourages hospitals to embrace the principles behind the 10 Steps to Successful Breastfeeding.[42] These steps aim to replace some hospital practices with an up-to-date approach based on scientific research.

Some steps are easily achieved by making very slight changes in hospital routine. Others are already in place in most hospitals.

Ten Steps to Successful Breastfeeding

- **Step 1:** Have a written breastfeeding policy that is routinely communicated to all healthcare staff.
- **Step 2:** Train all healthcare staff in skills necessary to implement this policy.
- **Step 3:** Inform all pregnant women about the benefits and management of breastfeeding.
- **Step 4:** Help mothers initiate breastfeeding about an hour after birth.
- **Step 5:** Show mothers how to breastfeed and how to maintain lactation, even if they have to be separated from their infants.
- **Step 6:** Give newborn infants no food or drink other than breast milk unless medically indicated.
- **Step 7:** Practice "rooming-in." Allow mothers and infants to remain together 24 hours a day.
- **Step 8:** Encourage breastfeeding on demand.
- **Step 9:** Give no artificial teats or pacifiers (also called *dummies* or *soothers*) to breastfeeding infants.
- **Step 10:** Foster the establishment of breastfeeding support groups and refer mothers to them on discharge from the hospital or clinic.

BACKGROUND NOTES (continued)

Further information about the Baby Friendly Hospital Initiative (BFHI) in the United States or Canada can be obtained from:

Wellstart International
Corporate Headquarters
4062 First Ave.
San Diego, CA 92103
or
Wellstart International
U.S. Committee for UNICEF
Baby-Friendly Hospital Initiative
4443 Pecan Valley Rd.
Nashville, TN 37218

Baby Friendly Hospital Initiative
UNICEF Canada
433 Mount Pleasant Road
Toronto, Ontario
M4S 2L8
Telephone: (416) 482-4444
Fax: (416) 482-8035

A MOTHER'S CHARTER

In England, a "Mothers' Charter" has been published to protect breastfeeding rights as part of the BFHI in Great Britain. To be breastfed is the healthiest start in life an infant can have. This Charter aims to protect a mother's right to breastfeed her baby.

Mother's Charter

A. It is your natural right to breastfeed your baby. It is your baby's natural right to be breastfed.

B. Your breast milk is tailor-made for your baby. It is specifically designed to nourish your baby, who usually needs no other form of baby food or drink in early infancy.

C. During your pregnancy, you should receive up-to-date information about the health benefits of breastfeeding both to you and to your baby. Exclusive breastfeeding to 4 months has been shown to provide the maximum health benefits to you both.

D. Your doctor or midwife should discuss breastfeeding fully with you during your prenatal care. Most breastfeeding problems can be prevented easily if you receive the right advice beforehand.

E. If you plan to have your baby in a hospital, ask to see a copy of the hospital's policy on breastfeeding. You need to be assured that you will receive help from skilled staff when you start to breastfeed.

F. Most mothers will want to be with their babies all the time. The hospital policy should clearly state that mothers and babies can be together 24 hours a day. This is called *rooming-in*.

G. You have a right to cuddle your baby right after delivery and to offer the important first breastfeeding. This is what your baby will instinctively want.

H. Healthcare staff should only advise that your baby be given artificial milk if it is medically necessary. In such cases, the reasons should be discussed with you in full before you give your consent.

I. If you and your baby have to be separated at any time, your baby should ideally receive your own expressed breast milk. Nurses or midwives will show you how to express your milk and maintain your supply.

J. Just like adults, babies like to drink different amounts at different times. Babies should be allowed to decide when to nurse and for how long. This type of baby-led feeding is often called *feeding on demand.*

K. Your right to breastfeed where and when you choose should never be questioned. No one should make you feel uncomfortable for doing what is best for your baby.

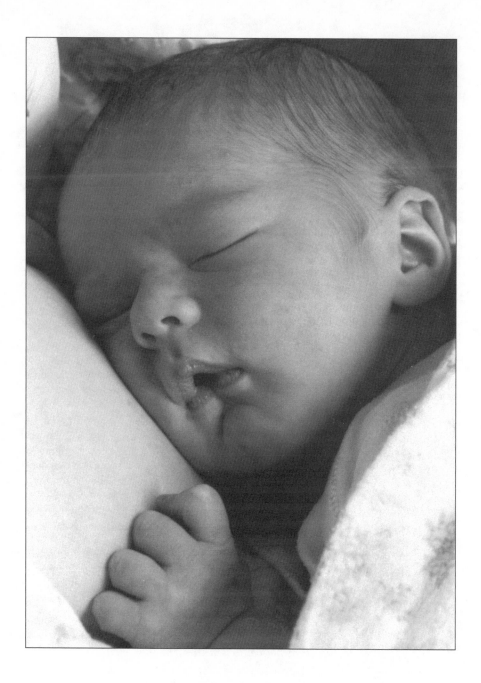

CHAPTER 4

Starting Out Together

Home Sweet Home

Going home after a hospital birth is the start of a completely new phase for you and your baby. Most of the time, going home is a positive step. Despite some nervousness, it is the time when you discover how it feels to have the responsibility of caring for a new baby. If you are a first-time mother, you may have to deal with many new experiences.

You may be relieved to return home, particularly if you have not found the hospital a relaxing place to breastfeed. For most women, going home is the start of getting to know their baby more intimately.

Debbie hated being in the hospital: *"The conflicting advice as the shifts changed. The antagonism from other women (who were bottle-feeding) who had been wakened by my baby. The midwives and nurses that put their fingers in my child's mouth. They gave bottles of water without my permission. They wouldn't let me sit alone in a room with my crying child at night; they told me to 'get my rest.' I was upset and humiliated by my lack of competence and frustrated by the lack of control."*

Once home, things got better and better for Claudette: *"I never timed the feedings, their duration or frequency. And I let Emily latch herself on, rather than pressing her on to my breast, just by holding her in the right position."*

Sandra found home the perfect place to enjoy getting to know her baby: *"Breastfeeding was heavenly with my first son. I felt so close to this little person whose eyes would try to focus on me in that wavering, in-and-out way. I knew I had to return to work within three months and Jacob and I spoiled each other rotten during that time. I loved being able to catch him before he got fussy. I loved the noises and slurps he made. I just loved the sensation of nursing. I carried him constantly, breastfed him on demand and hardly ever put him down. You can do that with a first child. I loved lying in bed with Jacob nursing between my husband and me. We felt so complete, just our own little world."*

After giving birth, you may find it hard to settle down and sleep. The excitement, satisfaction and likely relief mean most women are on an "emotional high" for some days after delivery. All this, plus the contact with other exuberant mothers and new babies can mean that most women return home pretty tired. The current trend is for you to be home one to two days after an uncomplicated delivery and about three days after a Cesarean birth.

Emotional and Practical Support

New mothers need plenty of emotional and practical support. In the very early days at home this support may be provided by your partner, close relatives or friends.

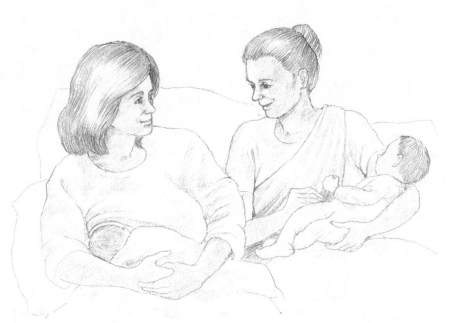

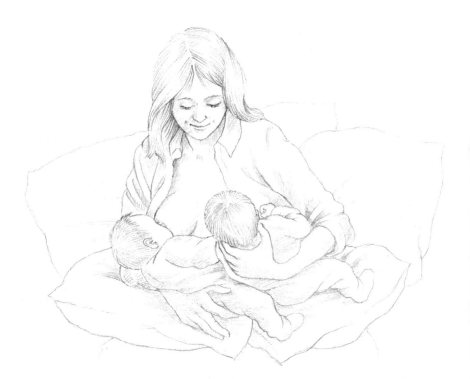

A recent survey of 115 U.S. mothers found that 75% of these women totally breastfed when their partner approved. But less than 10% breastfed if their partner either disapproved or was indifferent. Your partner, then, can be very influential. But it may be hard for some partners to learn how they can best contribute. Sometimes they can get it completely wrong, as Lois found out: *"Peter gave Tessa a bottle during that first night at home. He didn't wake me when she cried, thinking that I needed the rest. By morning I had badly engorged breasts with blocked ducts. I was terribly angry and felt useless. I also resented Tessa seeming to be content with a bottle. I felt even more determined not to give up breastfeeding."*

Other women may need their husbands' strength of purpose. Ann Marie's husband gave her just the support she needed: *"I feel the biggest influence was Ivan, my husband. Without his support, I think it would have been hard for me to keep breastfeeding Thomas. Ivan supported me during my emotional outbursts of self-doubt and let me know he believed in me. The whole picture would be totally different if at two o'clock in the morning he had wanted me to give Thomas a bottle."*

For many women, the positive attitude and good memory of their partner can translate into some valuable practical suggestions offered just at the right time. Moira's husband, Bob, reminded her of something they had learned: *"When my milk came in, my breasts were very full, so Lucy could not latch on. I was very emotional at the time—tired and frustrated at not being able to get my hungry baby fed. Thankfully my husband was thinking clearly. He remembered some points from the prenatal classes. He gently suggested I try changing the feeding position or have a shower to help relieve some of the pressure on my breasts."*

Some men may be able to provide more practical help than others, like Lois' partner: *"Peter became an expert on breast massage. He did this with dedication and good humor, without embarrassment, gently and tirelessly every three hours or so for three days. Without his very special support, I'm sure I would have developed mastitis and probably given up."*

The 1990 Infant Feeding Survey[1] found that 74% of women who were still breastfeeding at six weeks had been breastfed themselves. This suggests that a woman who has herself breastfed might be a positive, supportive role model for the new mother. Mothers and mothers-in-law are often there to help at home and give support after the baby is born, as Nicola found: *"My mother-in-law stayed with us for 10 days after the birth. She had breastfed all five of her babies. She was very supportive, never giving advice unless I directly asked for it."*

Other female relatives and friends who have breastfed may also offer support and encouragement. Elaine found the experiences of her sister-in-law invaluable: *"I had a visit when David was a week old from Sally, who was breastfeeding her seven-month-old son Hal. She suggested that I try Lansinoh® ointment to soothe my nipple soreness. She lent me some and it helped. Sally also pointed out that I could try to nurse David lying in bed, which was awkward at first with the [breast] shields, but I managed. What a difference that made! I could hardly feel him suck. So the next time I tried to take the shield off once the milk had let down, and I managed a pain-free latch. I was so relieved. At last I could really enjoy breastfeeding."*

Gail found talking with friends and relatives who had breastfed very useful: *"I was relieved to hear that other people had also had very painful nipples and still managed to continue nursing. A friend also showed me a nursing position that helped her but looked strange. But it worked. I leaned over the baby and dangled the breast into his mouth!"*

Patricia sought out other breastfeeding mothers: *"I remember needing reassurance that it was not unusual for the actual feeding times to increase. And for the times between feedings to decrease as the day progressed. Also, for the pattern and timing of feedings to vary on an almost-daily basis. This reassurance came from my sister-in-law and a friend, who had both breastfed their children, and from meeting with friends I'd made during the prenatal classes, who were also breastfeeding. The mutual support of the friends with babies of the same age as Lucy definitely made the first few months of breastfeeding and motherhood easier."*

After partners, mothers, mothers-in-law and female friends, health providers are also sources of support. Your healthcare practitioner can refer you to a professional lactation consultant. Such support is covered by many insurance plans. Lactation support may also be available through some Ministries of Health in Canada. (For contact information, see page 225). If you do not have insurance that covers lactation support, you may still contact La Leche League. La Leche League International has breastfeeding support groups throughout the United States and Canada. Their services are free. La Leche League leaders are specially trained mothers who are experienced at breastfeeding. La Leche League's 24-hour hotline is: 1-800-LA LECHE. You can call this number for immediate help with breastfeeding problems, or for the La Leche League support group nearest you. If the toll-free number is busy, call La Leche League at 1-847-519-0035 in the United States. In Canada, contact La Leche League at 1-613-448-1842 or at 1-514-747-9127 in Quebec. You will be referred to the La Leche League group nearest you.

In the United States, if you have Medicaid health insurance (Medi-Cal in California), you can also contact the Women, Infants and Children (WIC) program for breastfeeding support. WIC is a free supplemental-feeding program for women with low incomes and their children. It is a national program run by the Department of Health and Human Services and the U.S. Department of Agriculture. WIC staff provide a great deal of support to breastfeeding mothers. They also provide food coupons to improve nursing mothers' diets. In the United States, contact your nearest WIC program by calling your county or state Public Health Department.

Sometimes asking for help quickly improves a situation, as Vanessa found out: *"Close to tears, I asked Jon, my husband, to call a La Leche League leader who lives nearby. She came over within minutes, and just her presence gave me some reassurance. She watched me position Rachel and confirmed that I was doing all the right things. She asked my permission to help get Rachel latched on. Then she gently stroked the breast to try and encourage the milk flow. After we talked the whole thing through, she suggested that maybe Rachel wasn't hungry. What a revelation! I was so reassured to have someone with me, telling me that I was doing all the right things."*

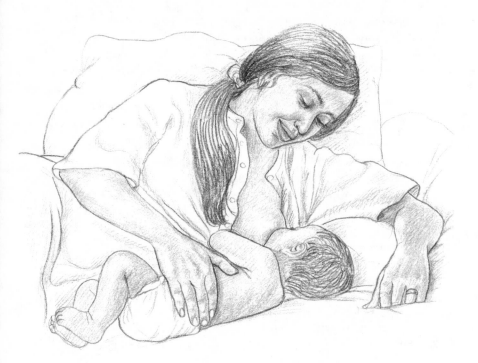

Elaine's experience with her lactation consultant was extremely positive: *"When my lactation consultant came over on the tenth day, my nipples were still sore. She was concerned about that, but enthusiastic about how well I had done so far. She got me to lie down on the bed and air them for 30 minutes after every feeding. I used plenty of towels to mop up my abundant milk supply, which seemed to want to let down every five minutes! Over the next few days, Joan, my lactation consultant, helped me to latch Jill on properly, without using the nipple shields, sitting on my bed with lots of pillows behind me to support my back. Without Joan's constant support, encouragement and enthusiasm, I think I might have just given up."*

During this early time at home, you may find it helps to turn to organizations such as La Leche League or WIC for guidance:

"Once I got home, my right nipple became sore. A friend who is a breast-feeding counselor came by. She put a cushion here, twisted the baby around 'football' style there, engineered a closer contact, a better latch—and voilá, no soreness."

"My lactation consultant also reassured me that I was doing all the right things. Hearing that from the expert really helped. Knowing she was on the end of the phone and knew about my situation was a real comfort."

Not all women are as lucky as those quoted above. The early weeks with a new baby can be a time when a mother may feel very alone. If your mother comes to stay to help you after your baby is born, she may have a different opinion about how things "should" be done. You may feel alone if you wish to follow childcare practices that are different from those most popular in your mother's day. Timing feedings and what to do when the baby cries seem to be the biggest problem areas.

Mary's mother-in-law and mother had very set ideas: *"My mother-in-law told me I should put her on the bottle because my milk was too thin. My mother couldn't advise me because she had not breastfed any of her babies. But I knew she felt I was spoiling Alex with on-demand feeding and trying to console her. She believed Alex was naughty and should be left to scream. I resented her idea that my problems were a result of my incompetence. I still felt I was doing the right thing."*

Isabel was under a lot of pressure to change the way she had started to do things: *"My husband had to travel for a few days, so my parents came and stayed. I did not feel good about being on my own all day and night. My parents had very rigid ideas about bringing up a baby. You fed it and then it went back to sleep and you rocked the cradle or walked up and down with the stroller until it did."*

You may feel torn between doing what your mother advises as best and doing what you feel you want to. It may depend on the relationship you already have. But usually some compromise can be reached. It may help to talk things through. Try to explain that you are not criticizing your mother because you do not want to do things the way she did.

You may feel lonely because family members are just not there to help you. Perhaps they are miles away. Or the burdens of earning a living give little space, time or energy for supporting a mother with a new baby.

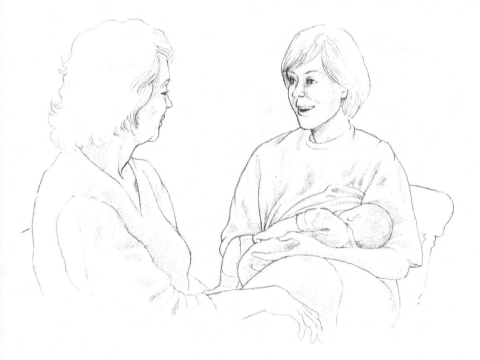

Mary was on her own much of the time and found it hard: *"I had no support from my family, partly because of distance. Thankfully, my husband was understanding, but he worked shifts and had a demanding job. I was often alone with a very cranky baby. I'd pace the floor all night rocking her while he was on night duty."*

Clearly good support, both practical and emotional, should be provided for all mothers. A recent survey in northeast Scotland[43] confirmed what many mothers know from experience. Tiredness and other physical or emotional problems are common after childbirth. Fifty-nine percent of mothers felt tired when their baby was two months old. And 61% said they weren't able to get as much rest as they needed. Half the mothers felt that they were not coping well when they first went home. And most of these still felt this way when their babies were eight weeks old. New mothers should receive support when they need it.[43] After giving birth, be selfish! Look after yourself. Relax and enjoy your baby as much as you can. "Normal life" will still be there in the months to come. The early months of babyhood will never return.

A Good Supply of Milk

Major concerns in the early weeks and months of breastfeeding may be: "Is my baby getting enough milk?" or "Is she or he gaining enough weight?" These concerns may come from a natural uncertainty as you get to know your baby. Or they may stem from worries raised by friends or relatives. Health providers sometimes question a mother's ability to breastfeed even before she has begun.

Beth remembers her fears when her daughter was weighed before leaving the hospital: *"Knowing I had to achieve a less-than 10% drop in birth weight in order to be allowed home was such pressure. Until my baby regained her birth weight, I was scared every time the nurse put her on the scales, in case she said I wasn't feeding her well."*

At 14 days, when weighed in the doctor's office, Anne-Marie's baby had lost weight and was well below his birth weight: *"At this stage, I needed a lot of reassurance and support. I appeared to be doing everything right but my baby was still losing weight. I felt very vulnerable to criticism and the 'Why don't you give him a bottle?' comments. Later I*

BACKGROUND NOTES

Weight guidelines

As a rough guide, the following weights may help you to judge your baby's weight gain or loss. It is worth trying to keep your baby in similar clothes when having him weighed. The differences in weight are fairly small. As you can see, what he is wearing can make a big difference. The weights are for a 6-week-old baby.

- Dry disposable diaper—approx. 1 oz.
- Wet disposable diaper—approx. 4 oz.
- Dry cloth diaper—approx. 5 oz.
- Wet cloth diaper—approx. 10 oz.
- Typical baby clothes: a sweater, sleepers, t-shirt, wet cloth diaper and plastic pants—approx. 1 lb. 3 oz.

learned that my husband had fielded a lot of these without telling me. I looked to my friends from the prenatal class who already had their babies and my doctor for support. And I depended a lot on the reassurance and support I got from my lactation consultant."

If you have not discussed early breastfeeding in terms of achieving a certain weight gain, a visit to a pediatrician's office, where there may be a lot of interest in the baby's weight, can come as quite a surprise, as it did to Ruth: *"I was alarmed when I took Laura to the clinic for the first time at 14 days, because they said she had lost weight. I was convinced that the scales were wrong. After we talked, the doctor advised me to wake Laura after five hours to nurse, because she wasn't getting enough feedings in 24 hours. I followed her advice and the next week she had gained eight ounces. The scales were correct. The doctor was happy. And there were never any other questions about her weight gain."*

Breastfeeding is, to some extent, a confidence game. You can do it if you *believe* that you can. Sadly, sometimes a poor weight gain is dealt with in ways that are likely to undermine your confidence *and* your milk supply.

Anne was looking forward to the first visit with the doctor. She and her husband dressed up for the occasion: *"Don and I had wondered how much weight Brad would have gained, but I remember saying: 'I wish his legs weren't quite so thin.' In fact, when Brad was weighed, we were all shocked to find that he had lost 14 ounces from his birth weight. One of the nurses glared at me and asked how many times a day I was feeding him. I told her five or six. They not only seemed very upset, but also gave me the feeling they thought that I had neglected Brad on purpose. Even as I am typing this, two years later, I feel upset about it."*

FEEDING FILE

How to boost your milk supply

- Eat as much as you need to satisfy your hunger. Spread out the food through the 24-hour day. Maybe have a snack whenever the baby nurses.
- Drink to quench your thirst. But don't force yourself to drink more than you want, because it can decrease your milk supply.
- Check the baby's position at the breast. If nursing hurts, seek help.
- Contact a lactation consultant or La Leche League leader for support.
- Take time to respond to your baby's need for sucking time: real "baby-led" feeding.
- Include extra, "not-asked-for" feeding sessions. It may be a good idea to wake your baby at night if she is sleeping for long periods.
- Cut out any other source of sucking. This includes a pacifier or bottled juice or water.
- Don't organize any major social events, just for the time being.

- Cut down on household chores. Accept any offers of practical help.
- Don't introduce a nipple shield or formula milk. These will interfere with your milk supply.
- Take the phone off the hook for a few hours each day and put your feet up.
- If you have other children, get baby-sitting help from other mothers or willing relatives.
- Express milk to increase stimulation for your breasts. Try *dual pumping*—pumping both breasts at once.
- Contact a lactation consultant or a La Leche League leader to learn about a good breast pump.
- La Leche League has leaflets on breastfeeding you may find useful. (See address on page 225).
- In the United States, your local WIC program may provide useful information. In Canada, your provincial or territorial Health Ministry may offer information or support.

Heather's experience was better, but still upsetting: *"I had a problem at the weekly weigh-in at the health center. After two visits that showed my daughter was not gaining the expected standard number of ounces, I was told I might have to supplement with a bottle. But two weeks later her weight gain had doubled and far exceeded the 'standard' increase."*

The definition of what is the "right" weight gain is itself open to question. Most of the growth charts in use are based on studies of mostly bottle-fed babies and were done in the 1950s.[44,45] Weight gain is not the only sign of a healthy baby. Is she alert and responsive? Is she happy most of the time? Does she have a good skin color (not very pale or grayish)? Does she produce plenty of "wet" diapers that don't smell? Are her stools mustard yellow? If so, she is almost certainly healthy.[34] Extra fluids can undermine your breastfeeding, both physically and emotionally.

FEEDING FILE

Cutting out complementary bottles

If you have been giving supplementary feedings of formula milk and want to cut these out, you should know that it is possible over time.

- If you are only giving one or two small bottles over 24 hours, be bold and cut them out. Increase the number of feedings you give your baby. Your breasts will produce more milk in response to the increased stimulation.

- Ask a lactation consultant or La Leche League leader to go through nursing positions with you. Check that your baby is nursing well.

- Try the tips for increasing your milk supply.

- If you are giving extra bottles at each feeding, it will take a little time to cut them out completely.

- Try putting an ounce less into each bottle.

- Offer the breast again after the bottle. The extra stimulation will help to boost your supply.

- Cut out one bottle at a time. Start with the one you give when you seem to have the most breast milk available. Make the change gradually, over a few days, to enable your breasts time to build up a supply.

- Once you have cut out one bottle, use the same strategy to cut out the others. Take your time and think positive. It can be done!

- Support from your family and friends will help, especially if your baby is a bit more cranky while your supply catches up with his needs.

In some cases, there may be a real need to boost your milk supply. The best action to take in that case will depend on your own circumstances.

Suzi's baby was happy and contented, but not very sleepy. He seemed to gain weight very slowly: *"I decided to increase the number and lengths of feedings, whether they were demanded or not. We spent many happy hours together nursing and I look back on this time with affection. After a while, his weight began to increase steadily. The test weighing stopped and to my relief he filled out nicely."*

Amy's little boy, Timothy, didn't gain weight very well and was fretful. She felt that she might be producing too little milk for him: *"I looked in my books and leaflets. They suggested resting more and forgetting about the housework. I began to eat well rather than dieting as I had begun to do to get rid of the extra weight. And I nursed more often. After a few weeks he was happier and began to gain more weight."*

Anne found her baby's doctor was extremely supportive: *"She told me that she had experienced very similar problems with her first baby. She was therefore able to understand only too well what I was going through. I was, and still am, grateful for her support at that time. She taught me about formula feedings, which Alan needed to get his weight up quickly. She encouraged me to continue to breastfeed as well, and to try to increase my milk supply in the hope of being able to drop bottle feedings."*

Maggie blames herself for her initial problems. But after some searching she found the support she needed: *"When he started to cry and it wasn't five hours since his last feeding, I would shove a pacifier in his mouth. Within a week he lost 1-½ pounds and my milk supply was nothing. The pediatrician told me I had lost my milk and should give him a bottle. I knew this was wrong, deep down, so I went to see my family doctor. She also told me I'd lost my milk and I would need to give him a bottle. In desperation and tears, my husband and I decided to give him a bottle. But it just didn't feel right. I wanted so badly to look like those happy breastfeeding pictures you see.*

"My husband encouraged me to call La Leche League. I called and a terrific woman came to my house within 30 minutes. She taught me so much. She gave me confidence I didn't have. I stopped giving him a pacifier when he cried and instead put him to my breast. I nursed him every hour for four days until I suddenly appeared engorged. My milk supply had increased. (I've since learned that you don't lose it, it just decreases.) Now when I hear people telling me to supplement with a bottle, I call my La Leche League leader and get my breastfeeding reality check."

It may help to know that some babies gain weight slowly on formula milk and have periods of unexplained crying too, as Linda found out: *"I was very sad to stop breastfeeding. I had failed and I didn't really know why. Despite being fully bottle-fed, my baby's weight gain was poor, less than half the average amount. He did vomit at each bottle-feeding, but I was told that was normal. Five weeks later, the weight gain was still poor. The pediatrician was worried and so my baby was admitted to the hospital for observation. I really felt he was not sick. He was too alert and taking a lot of interest in his surroundings. At the end of the week, the weight gain was only two ounces. They could not find anything wrong. After doing various tests, we were sent home. At around 2-½ months, his weight gain became normal. I cannot understand why,*

*when so much emphasis is put on weight gain, that family circum-
stances aren't considered. Throughout this experience, I pointed out
that neither I nor my husband tend to put on weight, yet we both eat
well. Both sets of grandparents are the same way. Surely genetics or
metabolism must have been a factor to consider."*

It's clearly important to look at each mother-and-baby pair on their
own. Weight gain should not be the only way to judge the "success" of
breastfeeding.

Growth Spurts

Behavioral changes during these early weeks of the baby's life do not
always mean that you are not producing enough milk for your baby. You
could simply be a little tense and your milk may not let down too well.

At five to seven weeks, many babies suddenly increase their demand
for milk. This is commonly called a "growth spurt." It may take you by
surprise. Your calm baby will suddenly ask to nurse more often. If you
continue to offer him the breast whenever he cries you will quickly

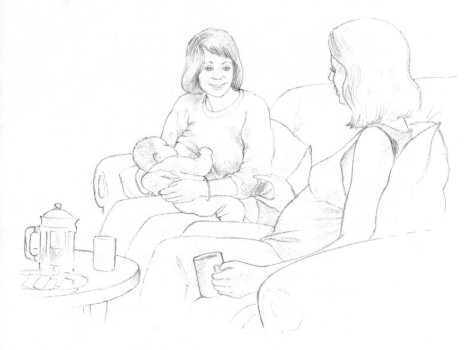

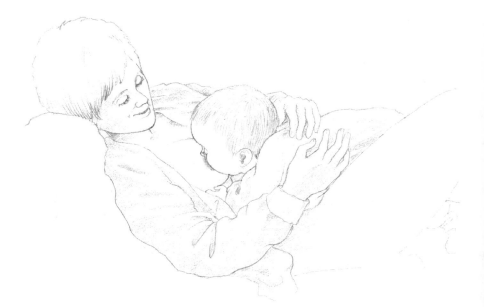

increase the amount of milk you have to match his new requirements. If you begin formula at this time, you will give breast milk a chance to increase to match your baby's new needs. Over 24 to 48 hours, your supply will increase to meet your baby's needs. He may continue nursing at this increased rate for a week or so, and then drop back to his previous pattern.

Elaine's patience and determination to continue breastfeeding helped her through a tense time: *"When David was five or six weeks old, he seemed to want to nurse more often during the evening and at night. One time he woke up at 11 in the evening, half an hour after I had put him down to sleep for what I thought was going to be the next three or four hours. I was exhausted and fed up. He was crying and kicking so I couldn't get him latched on for at least 20 minutes, which just made things worse. My breasts felt empty. My nipples were sore and I was convinced I had nothing left to give him. My husband suggested we give David a bottle of milk. At that moment I would have loved to have done that—but we didn't have any in the house.*

"We took turns pacing the floor with a crying baby. He would doze off for 10 minutes, but if we tried to put him down, he would start crying again. I made myself a sandwich and a cup of decaf coffee, in an effort to "make milk." Half an hour later I tried to latch him on again. This time, success! I practiced relaxation techniques and 'thought milk,' which helped my prickly let-down sensation. David nursed for half an

hour. This showed me how such an emotional situation, filled with frustration, pain and tiredness, plus a lack of information, could have led to me bottle-feeding."

Too Much Milk

At the other end of the spectrum, some mothers and babies have trouble with too much milk. This can also be frustrating, particularly because many people may not recognize how awkward it can be. Joy suffered

---

FEEDING FILE

Tips to help with too much milk

- Nurse your baby whenever he wants to in the early days.

- It may take up to about 10 weeks to balance the amount of milk you produce with what your baby needs.

- It may be OK to offer only one breast per feeding, after a while.

- Rub gently around the areola with ice cubes wrapped in a washcloth to help the nipple stand out.

- Place a cold washcloth on your breasts.

- You may need to "think milk;" that is, get your milk flowing and release some of the foremilk before bringing the baby to the breast. Try to do this without using a pump. A pump will only add to the stimulation and may increase the amount of milk you make.

- Nurse your baby lying down, with her on top of you. You may have to support the baby's forehead. This is sometimes called *upside-down gravity feeding.*

- Be prepared to "mop up" excess milk while nursing.

- It may be possible to collect the milk flowing from one breast while your baby is nursing from the other breast. Store it for future use or donate it to a milk bank.

- To reduce the milk flow from a breast, press gently into the breast with the heel of your hand.

- If milk flows from both breasts when you don't want it to, fold your arms in front of you and gently press inwards.

- A bra that enables you to nurse with one breast at a time is most helpful. Breastpads can be held in place on one side while you nurse from the other.

- You may want to use plastic-backed breast pads if you are going out and need to protect your clothes. Do not use them all the time, though, because they prevent your skin from "breathing" and can cause soreness.

- Keep a spare blouse with you, just in case.

from an enormous supply and soon felt she had to stop breastfeeding: *"I was flooded with milk. I think the best way to describe it is—it was like someone pouring two cups of warm water down my front every hour. I gave up after two weeks because the flooding didn't get better. I was scared to go out because I couldn't control the leakage."*

For others, like Evelyn, the flow was not quite so overwhelming: *"I was surprised by the amount of milk I had. For the first four weeks or so I was soaked with milk. I stocked the freezer with bottles. I thought I would never be able to go out because my clothes got drenched every time my baby was due for a feeding. After a while, it all worked out."*

Practical information often helps, as Cath discovered: *"I turned to my lactation consultant for help. She listened and supported me. She suggested that I try to express a little foremilk just before nursing, to take away the first gush of milk. I also tried different feeding positions, including lying flat on my back with my baby on top of me. But it took about nine weeks before she was able to nurse in comfort."*

There is often too much milk in the first few weeks. The relationship between the amount of milk the baby requires and the amount produced by the breasts is delicately balanced. The right amount often becomes established during the first six to seven weeks, but may take about 10 weeks. There are clearly exceptions to this. You will likely learn your own ways to enable you and your baby to breastfeed. It is also good to remember that wearing drip-catching breast shields to collect extra milk can often make the problem worse. They put constant pressure on your milk ducts, so you keep on leaking.

Growing Confidence

Ideally, you will gently learn about yourself in your new role by interacting with your baby: cuddling, bathing and feeding her. As days and weeks pass, you will begin to feel more comfortable and confident with both the practical aspects of babycare and the emotions that go with caring for a new human being.

Sophie describes how breastfeeding helped her build confidence as a mother: *"I was still trying to gain self-esteem as a new mother, trying to understand the intensity and variety of feelings I had towards my baby. Love and satisfaction could be swiftly followed by feelings of entrapment*

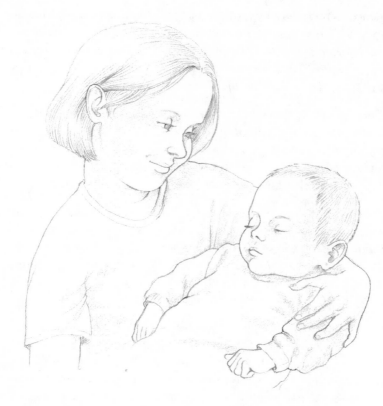

and irritability. Then I felt selfish for wanting my own life and guilt and remorse when things went wrong. To the outside world, I was doing great. But I felt like I was failing at motherhood, doing a bad job. I was confused. Once breastfeeding was established, I felt it was one of the few things I did right as a mother."

If your natural development of confidence is interrupted by unkind, undermining comments, you may feel demoralized. It can be hard to choose to keep on breastfeeding when your belief in your ability has been shaken. At best, you will be able to turn to supportive relatives and friends to help you through. There could be moments, though, when, despite this support, you feel breastfeeding is an uphill struggle. It may help to talk to a lactation consultant. She will have breastfed her own babies and will remember the panicky feelings that come when things do not seem to be going too well. Talking with an understanding lactation consultant could be all you need to get through a bad time.

Confidence is recognized as a very special component of the breast-feeding experience. It is an important ingredient for successful breast-feeding and something women would like to share with each other.

Cindy comments: *"If I could give a mother anything, it would be confidence—the confidence to relax. The confidence to know that she really is the person who knows what is best for her baby. And the confidence to sift through all the 'advice' she will get from all sorts of crazy sources."*

Jill remembers: *"I learned to take everyone's comments about the quality and quantity of my milk with a large pinch of salt. But it took me about eight or nine weeks to be really confident that I could nurse him. If I could give any advice, it would be* believe in yourself. *If you really want to breastfeed, you can!"*

Experience brings a relaxed attitude, as Melissa discovered: *"This time, as an older mom with 16 years as a childbirth educator under my belt, I'm confident enough to do things my way. I'm much more aware of the need to eat and drink plenty and rest and let other things wait. A supportive husband who definitely thinks 'breast is best' makes it so much easier. He, too, is more mature, and even more encouraging this time around. And I'm pleased to have the chance to show my elder daughter that breastfeeding is good and normal and possible."*

Your confidence grows as the baby grows. Mothers often experience enormous pride and happiness in the success of the relationship they have from breastfeeding their babies. Sandra is sure that breastfeeding her baby has made all the difference in their relationship: *"I dreaded the birth of my third baby. I was so unhappy at the prospect of having another baby to care for. The unfolding of my love for her was completely bound to our breastfeeding together. Through breastfeeding, my love for her grew. By breastfeeding I supplied all her needs myself. I was so proud of myself and my lovely new baby, I went on to breastfeed her for 11 months."*

Pam found feeding Scott an incredibly rewarding experience: *"I clearly remember gushes of pride and self-congratulation when I looked at him at four months. I thought to myself, 'This is all, every single cell of his body, due to my hard work. Amazing.' As my confidence grew, it felt great just to throw away the books and do what I felt was right for me and Scott."*

Perhaps there should be a TV commercial about this way to happiness and self-fulfillment. Is it something that breastfeeding women have been reluctant to discuss? We live in a culture where breastfeeding a small baby in a restaurant might be frowned upon. It is not surprising that those who continue and enjoy breastfeeding are reluctant to talk about the emotional satisfaction they receive from the relationship that develops between themselves and their babies.

Some people are too ready to dismiss a mother's satisfaction as some-how not important. There is plenty of information available about breastfeeding's health benefits to you and your baby, which has been well researched. Sadly, we do not hear so much about the positive feelings women have about their capacity to breastfeed, nor how good a positive breastfeeding experience can be for self-esteem.[46] There must be psychological and emotional benefits for your baby as well, in having an attentive, responsive, satisfied mother offering food and comfort from her breast.

A Flexible Lifestyle

Several years ago, we were expected to feed small babies on a four-hour schedule. Between the feedings, new mothers were encouraged to get on with the household chores. In recent times, couples have been told to demand-feed their baby. This means feeding your baby when he is hungry and not "by the clock." Sometimes it is called *natural* or *baby-led feeding*. In the early days, giving the baby the breast whenever he cries will encourage your breasts to develop a generous milk supply.

It can be difficult to think about this before the baby comes. The concept of the baby "demanding" to be fed may not feel right to you. After all, many couples go through pregnancy assuring, or maybe convincing, themselves that a baby will not change their comfortable lifestyle. Many new parents do not want their lives altered too much by the arrival of the baby. Questions such as "How often does demand feeding mean?" "When will the baby go to sleep?" "Will there be times when life can get back to normal?" may go through your mind. This part of baby care is a step into the unknown.

Each baby is a unique person with his or her own special nursing needs, as Barbara came to accept: *"I never knew, from one day to another, when she would be awake or asleep, or when she would want to nurse.*

FEEDING FILE

Your new roles as parents

During the first few weeks, nursing your baby may seem to take over your life. There may seem to be little time or energy left for anything else. You have all just become a family and it is important to give each other time to adjust to your new roles.

A role for your partner

- Ask your partner to "field" unwanted visitors and telephone calls.
- Purchase a "baby sling" carrier and encourage your partner to take your baby out in it. In colder months, a ride in the car or well-wrapped in a stroller may work equally well—and give you a break.
- Ask your partner to give a bottle of expressed breast milk for a late evening feeding so that you can get more sleep.

Make time for each other

- Try to spend time with each other. Becoming parents involves major changes in how you see yourselves. There will be lots to talk about. Try to keep each other in touch with how you feel as individuals and as a couple.
- If you would like to go out together without your baby, get a well-known and trusted person to baby-sit. You could leave a bottle of expressed breast milk. Or breastfeed just before leaving and as soon as you return.
- Retain and value your sense of humor.
- Express "tender loving care" regularly.

At first I found this hard to take. I was always not having a shower or not starting to write a letter because she might wake up. Then, of course, she would sleep for a long time and I wouldn't have accomplished anything. In time, I got used to doing things in short bursts, with a longer stretch now and then. Breastfeeding was an advantage, because when she woke up I could nurse her immediately. I didn't have to make time for fixing bottles and sterilizing. I spent countless hours nursing her, daydreaming or reading a book."

Sometimes it is hard to imagine what it will really be like to breastfeed and, like Yolanda, you may need time to adjust: *"I never thought what a commitment breastfeeding would be until I did it. If your baby has no particular routine, you have to be around 24 hours a day to nurse. I have vivid memories of trying to do Christmas shopping when my daughter was 3-½ months old. I'd phone home every half hour to make sure she wasn't screaming for food. I expressed milk for her into a bottle, which she would drink if she was hungry. But I also found that if I was away for more than three or four hours at a time, my breasts would become really full and uncomfortable."*

Ruth had the memory of nursing her first daughter to encourage her: *"For the first three or four months of Mary's life, I never knew where I was with nursing. No two days were the same. I never felt I could leave Mary. I didn't know when she would need to nurse. There were times when I felt resentful, like a nursing machine. I felt tied and desperately tired. At those times, I could understand a woman wanting to give up breastfeeding. But I was determined to continue. I feel that the memory of nursing Laura successfully encouraged me to keep going."*

Sally followed her baby's lead: *"After the first few weeks, he'd nurse mostly at about three hours. Then his pattern changed a little, and sometimes he'd go four hours, sometimes only two. After a while, I stopped looking at the clock and was much happier then. After all it didn't really matter if we were both happy."*

In order to maintain the baby's milk supply, your breasts need to be stimulated quite often. Luckily, small babies enjoy their time at the breast. Giving your baby free access to your breasts ensures that plenty of milk will be there for him. Sometimes he may take a small "snack" from the breasts. At other times he will want to spend much longer nursing, taking both the foremilk and the fat-rich hindmilk. Adults are this way, too: sometimes we prefer a sandwich, other times we'd like a three-course meal. A baby's stomach is very small, so it can't hold very much. During a 24-hour period, your baby will take both "short" and "long" feedings. He will regulate his own appetite, taking just what he needs when he needs it. Over the weeks, some babies do seem to develop their own patterns of nursing. You will begin to recognize these patterns, as these mothers did:

"My first baby nursed all the time throughout his 12-hour days, but slept through the night from an early age. My second nursed so quickly and so little (more or less every four hours) that I thought there was something wrong. Number three was like number two."

"Alex nursed frequently. It always seemed easier to nurse her than to find other ways to distract her. At about six weeks, I remember a visit from a friend with her first baby, born a few days before Alex. Her son nursed once while I managed about three feedings."

Few babies adopt a definite, repeating pattern that can be relied upon. Each day could be different. Your baby may need more food or comfort today than he did the day before. If you expect him to be the same today as he was yesterday, you will be surprised.

There could be times in a day when it seems as though your baby does not really know what he wants. You can try lots of different ways to comfort him only to find that nothing works for very long. These are the frustrations felt during the early days as mother and baby learn to understand one another. But as days pass into weeks, most parents do begin to understand and interpret their baby's cries quite well.

Demand feeding can work both ways. You can encourage your baby to nurse when the baby has not asked to do so. For example, if you wish to leave your baby or visit a place where you do not expect it to be easy for you to breastfeed, you could nurse the baby beforehand so that he is full while you are away.

Nursing and Sleeping

Small babies do not notice the difference between night and day—there is no day and night in the womb. In fact, many pregnant women find that their baby becomes active when they settle down for a night's sleep. For the baby, nursing must occur whenever it is needed, day or night. As your milk supply builds to meet the baby's needs, your breasts will become extremely uncomfortable if your baby does not nurse. The milk-making hormone prolactin is present in your bloodstream in greater amounts at night. So night nursing is really good for building up and keeping a good supply of milk. Responding quickly to the cries of your baby and keeping her close to you will make it easiest for you to nurse. In time, she will pick up cues from you and learn that night hours are not for socializing. The time and frequency of night feedings is very individual.

Some mothers, like Lucy, find that their babies sleep through the night at a very early age: *"She slept through the night from about 11 o'clock to six in the morning from four weeks old, and her night gradually got longer."*

Having a baby who sleeps through the night can cause problems, though, as Helen found: *"At around eight months, bedtime became easier. But he still wanted fairly frequent feedings, usually every couple of hours. Although the last feeding was around eight in the evening, by 11 o'clock I would be getting uncomfortably full. So before I went to bed, I would lift the baby out of the crib, nurse him and put him back. It was as if he had not been disturbed."*

Some babies take a lot longer to settle into a clear distinction of daytime and nighttime behavior, like Elaine's baby: *"David kept nursing frequently throughout the night. I think that I would have been concerned about him if I had not had Jenny as a role model. Her baby nursed all night and there was clearly nothing wrong with him."*

Constant night waking is tiring and can be stressful. Some couples accept it easily and adjust their own sleeping patterns to allow for the tiredness they may experience. They may, perhaps, go to bed a little sooner, or sometimes take a nap during the day. It seems that some parents believe the waking is linked to the way they feed their baby. It is true that breast milk is more easily digested than formula milk. Therefore, some breastfed babies will ask to nurse frequently.

For Jane, this fact came to her attention too late: *"No one told me that breast milk digests more quickly than bottled milk, so a baby is less likely to sleep through the night. I was totally fed up with getting up at least once every night and never knowing how long it would be till I woke up to a baby's crying. I felt chained to the baby and my boobs. We could never be more than three hours apart."*

Babies fed on formula milk may go longer between feedings. But don't assume that a baby will simply change his feeding needs if he stops breastfeeding. Some women introduce formula believing and hoping that if they do so their baby will "go longer between feedings" or "sleep all night." Sometimes the first few formula feedings may have that effect, because the baby's stomach is not used to the different makeup of the milk. Often, the amount of formula will need to be increased to maintain the effect. In some cases, formula milk has no effect on the baby's sleeping habits. And for some, it can lead to an upset stomach and more nighttime troubles.

There is no guarantee that formula will change your baby's habits, but Colette says she has been tempted to try it: *"From my completely random and unscientific study of friends and acquaintances with young babies, I am convinced that bottle-fed babies do sleep better. Of course there are bottle-fed babies who are bad sleepers, but nearly all of the good sleepers are bottle-fed. I know the reason is that formula milk is said to be harder to digest than breast milk. The result is that the bottle-fed baby lasts longer between feedings. I also know that breastfeeding counselors would argue that breast milk is so much better for a baby than formula milk that all the broken nights are worthwhile. After eight months of sleepless nights, I am not convinced!"*

Learning to Be Flexible

One challenge of parenting is to adjust to the changing ways of children as they grow and develop, regardless of how they are fed. People may live fairly orderly lives before becoming parents. Adjusting to the flexible nature of a baby may not be easy. Perhaps the most difficult change to accept is the feeling of not being in control of how a day will turn out. Many adults strive to "be in control" of their lives, perhaps thinking that being in control is the route to coping successfully with life. Babies, on the other hand, are not in control of anything. They express their needs as and when they occur, quite loudly at times. While caring for a new baby, you may begin to wonder when you will manage to be "in control" of the baby and your lives again.

Parents of older children acknowledge their children as totally separate individuals very easily. They know from experience that they do not "control" their children. Perhaps it would be easier all around if it were accepted as soon as a baby is born that parents are not meant to "control" their babies. This would save the heartache and struggles connected with parents determined to "get the baby into a routine" long before it is possible or appropriate to do so.

Sunita would be the first to say that having children has taught her a lot about basic human psychology: *"After all, who says babies and toddlers don't need to be fed at night? Do we have telepathic insight into what our children need? Are we dictating our children's behavior? Or do we allow them to have minds of their own? Surely they are the best judge of what they need and don't need. A fulfilled need is one that goes away. Children are little for such a short time of our lives, I believe we owe it to them to satisfy those needs."*

Getting to know your baby and trying to learn how to respond to his needs, free from the expectations of routine or the pressure of trying to be in control, can be a joyful and fulfilling experience, as Carly agrees: *"I'm kind of a breastfeeding junkie. At the end of a long day (and some days are very long!), my baby lies soothed in my arms as she strokes my skin. Her eyes close and she becomes totally satisfied and peaceful. I stroke her brow and her soft chubby cheeks and think I know why this relationship is the ultimate nurturing experience."*

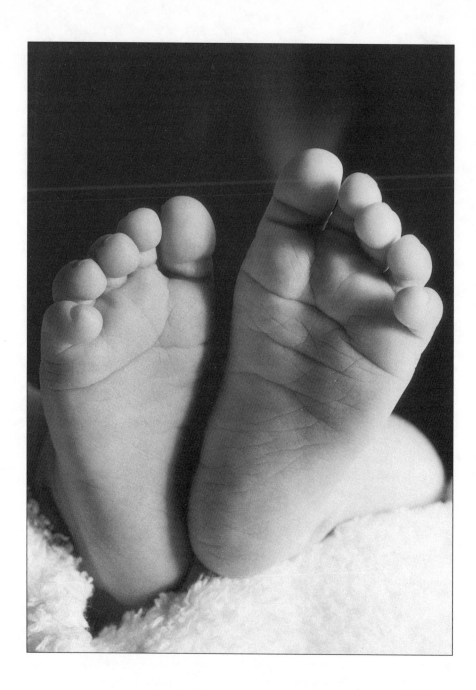

CHAPTER 5

Stepping Out with Confidence

Getting Around with Your Baby

After the first few weeks of learning to breastfeed, most mothers look forward to resuming a more "normal" life. This means you will need to be able to nurse your baby in comfort when strangers are around and when you are out of the house. For some women, the first hurdle will be nursing in front of visitors in your own home.

Judy's first experience of how embarrassed other people may feel led to a lot of confusion: *"The meal was simmering on the stove and need-ed an occasional stir. My baby son decided he wanted to be nursed, so I offered him my breast—at which point, the guests all decided to try and find something to read on the wall to divert their gaze. They were relieved to realize they could go and look around the backyard. My hus-band followed with bewilderment, wondering what had caused the stampede. I was left with no one to talk to, and a meal that might burn.*

"At this point I should explain that my baby, although able to breast-feed, was not able to create much suction. The slightest movement I made would take him off the breast and disturb his feeding. Finally, my first son returned to find out if I was all right. I have to admit to feeling more than upset. I asked him to get my husband to watch the meal. Then there was a crazy scene with the relatives outside, me inside breastfeeding, my husband cooking. When the feeding was finished, I put the little one to bed. As soon as my relatives realized I was fully cov-ered, they made a bee-line back to the house and the sofas."

For some women, there seem to be two main areas of concern. First, "Will I be able to do it?" which could be translated as, "Can I bare my breasts in public?" And second, "What will other people's reactions be?" which could be translated as, "Will I be embarrassed?"

Breastfeeding in public was a big concern to Lesley at first: *"I found it was extremely helpful to be with women from my childbirth class who were also breastfeeding. My first experiences were very positive and relaxed. When Laura and I ventured into the big, wide world, it wasn't a problem. Discretion was always my motto. But no way was I nursing Laura in public bathrooms. I quickly learned the 'baby-friendly' stores with the right facilities and planned my errands around them."*

When it came to nursing her baby in front of other people, Angela did sometimes feel a bit self-conscious: *"But I also hoped that I was maybe in a small way helping break down barriers for others. The more women are seen nursing in public, the more acceptable it becomes, as long as they are sensitive to other people's feelings. Maybe I was also proud of my breasts at last."*

Sometimes older friends or members of the family can help you feel confident about breastfeeding away from your own home. Tracy was pleased to find this was the case: *"I can recall visiting my grandparents-in-law with my first child, about six weeks old. They were horrified when my husband suggested I go upstairs to nurse her. I was really glad that they were so supportive. (They are both in their 80s.)"*

Sadly, not all grandparents are so supportive, as Tani discovered: *"At Katy's feedings I was supposed to go to the back bedroom to spare Grandpa any embarrassment. But Katy nursed frequently in the evenings, and it was lonely there. I felt stigmatized. We did reach a compromise—I was allowed in the family room with my chair turned to the wall! I am surprised that I still feel angry about this attitude."*

It's likely you will not feel any anxiety at all about nursing outside your own home. Once you have established breastfeeding, you may find it more stressful not to respond to your baby's cries for food. You may also feel the sensations that come with letting your milk down. This is a reflex action that is an efficient means of readying milk for your baby. The baby's cry triggers the reflex, which responds by letting down milk. Knowing you can calm your baby simply and quickly means that you may want to breastfeed when you are out and about, even if you might have hesitated previously. As any new parents know, a crying baby is likely to be more noticeable than one quietly enjoying his feeding.

Janet was always a very private feeder: *"My experiences outside are few. Once I nursed in the entrance of a restaurant in an interstate service station. (I couldn't afford to eat there, but we weren't asked to leave.) Once I nursed in a field after a so-called fun run. I didn't nurse away from home very often unless I was in someone's house. No one ever suggested that I stop or do it elsewhere, even when I was in a nonbreastfeeding house. I would have been mortified if they had! It used to cross my mind . . . what if someone asks me to move? What will I do? Nothing, it turns out, because no one ever did glare or complain. Which makes me realize that lots of babies are being breastfed out there. But because it is easy and calm and quiet, no one notices."*

For mothers of twins, discreet breastfeeding may not be an option, as Tricia describes: *"Next came going out. (You can't remain a hermit because you've got twins!) Friends would invite us over for meals and we'd request a sofa and two pillows. It was usually—Hi, how are you?*

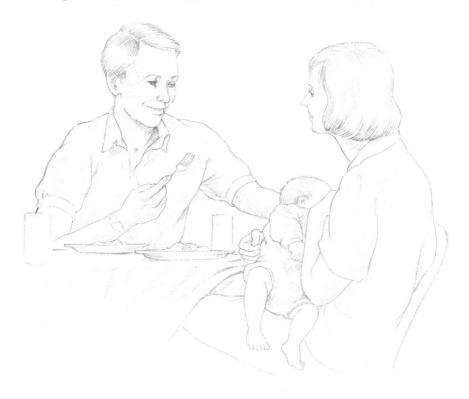

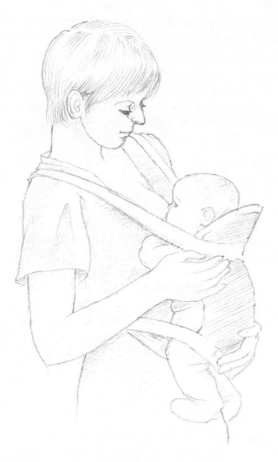

and Where's the sofa, you don't mind, do you? Up with the blouse and out with the boobs! There was no way you could be modest or discreet until the babies were latched on. Then, possibly, you could pull the blouse down. Going shopping was fit in between feedings. There really aren't too many places you can breastfeed twins in public, unless I nursed them separately. But that would throw them off their routine for the rest of the day. We took a trip during the period I was breastfeeding. Flights don't always fit into babies' schedules, so we used a bottle during the day. We juggled those around flying times (the twins were six months old). On our vacation, we rented a small minivan with a large back seat. I made myself comfortable, and away we went."

Many mothers find they are able to breastfeed whenever and wherever they need, without it ever being a problem. All you need is confidence, as these mothers testify.

Stepping Out with Confidence

.... *91*

Colette wonders whether her lack of embarrassment was related to her age. Being older gave her more confidence perhaps: *"In our area, we have very few nursing facilities in public places. So Luke was nursed in the car, in parks, in restaurants—wherever. No one ever asked me to stop. I even nursed him during take-off on a plane and on a train. I think most people would rather see a baby nurse than hear it screaming its head off. I'm sure a few people (mostly men) looked the other way when they saw me plug Luke in. I don't blame them. It can be hard to know what to do in a situation like that. So little public breastfeeding is seen these days that it isn't surprising (but too bad) that people can be fazed by it."*

Louise and her husband thrive on the ease of breastfeeding. Louise suggests: *"My one tip is not to ask if it's OK. The one time I asked if I could nurse him I was told 'No'! My husband and I also do a lot of hiking, so breastfeeding is perfect. I've nursed out on hiking trails plenty of times."*

Nursing in public came easily to Sheila: *"I nursed Helen everywhere. Standing in a parking lot, cafes, airports, on the bus, on a bench downtown. Always discreetly, wearing lift-up T-shirts, not button-up clothes. Sometimes I would be talking to someone who would suddenly realize I was nursing Helen. When she reached seven months, Helen would pull away too much to be discreet. By then it wasn't a problem, though, because I would rarely be out for her few feedings."*

Jill has other words of encouragement: *"I would like to say to other mothers, don't be afraid to nurse your baby in public. It can be done very discreetly. In fact, go out as much as you can while your baby only needs milk. It gets much harder and messier while they are being weaned. I've nursed in all sorts of places. I never asked permission. And I've never sat and nursed in a lounge or a public restroom. I don't think of nursing a baby as something to be hidden away. The reaction of other people (if any) has always been neutral or positive."*

It's possible to nurse your baby anywhere, as Dina proved: *"I can't remember ever thinking, 'No, not here.' I wasn't a militant who was determined to breastfeed to prove a point or anything. I just never found myself in a place where I couldn't nurse my son discreetly. So I nursed him wherever I was. The only time I ever used any special facility was in a baby store or a drugstore when I was out shopping in the cold. In nice weather, I've nursed Gilbert outdoors—on a bus bench on a sidewalk. I was chatting with a friend the whole time, and I don't think that any-*

one except us knew I was nursing. I've nursed him in parks, on beaches, in restaurants at home and on vacation, on a ferry, in bars, on an airplane, in a forest. I've even nursed him more than once while giving a lecture. I nursed him on a hospital gurney while waiting for a scan. And I never felt, or was made to feel, uncomfortable doing it."

Others' reactions to seeing women breastfeed in public places can be interesting. Displaying breasts as sexual objects of desire and arousal seems to be fine. Look at all the current magazines and movies. Meanwhile, we occasionally hear of a mother, quietly breastfeeding her baby, being asked to leave the local department store.What's wrong with this picture?

During a talk given at the 1995 National Childbirth Trust Annual Conference in England, Elizabeth Bradley, a child psychiatrist and psychoanalyst, explained that negative reactions to women breastfeeding their babies may result from largely unconscious memories of a poor breastfeeding relationship with a person's own mother. As a result, such people may be almost completely out of touch with the needs of

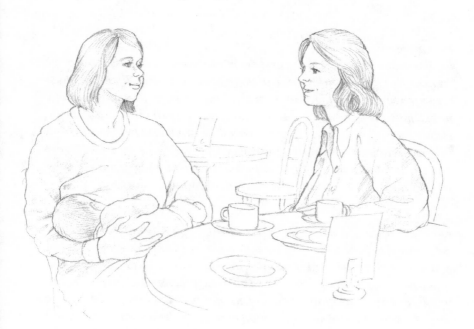

the baby for the comfort derived from his mother's breast. Conversely, those who feel comfortable seeing a baby at the breast are in touch with the needs of the baby. It may be that they have their own good memories of breastfeeding.

Is it fair that a breastfeeding woman should be burdened with the worries of other people's reactions to her nursing her baby? When one woman at a prenatal class suggested there could be adverse reactions to a woman breastfeeding in public, a young man in the room responded strongly by saying that other people's feelings were their business and their problem. They were not going to affect how he and his partner were going to feed their baby. His confidence may have helped his family experience a positive breastfeeding experience.

A breastfed baby can travel easily because his nutritional needs can be met simply as long as he is not too far away from his mother.

Lulu discovered how easy it is to travel with a breastfed baby: *"I took my daughter along to a few parties and social events. I was able to breastfeed her on these occasions without attracting any adverse comments or looks. One time a person did not even believe I was breastfeeding her, we were so discreet. My daughter was so quiet and peaceful that he was convinced she was simply asleep in my arms.*

"When my daughter was nine months old, my partner and I took her on a month-long, around-the-world trip. The fact I was still breastfeeding her really helped. She became fussy now and then during the trip, due to the changing time zones and sleeping in different beds. Putting her to my breast was the best way to give her comfort and help her feel secure. By breastfeeding, we never had to worry about bringing formula milk with us, sterilizing bottles or finding sterile water. This trip certainly reinforced my belief in the positive effects of breastfeeding. I think many women are wary of breastfeeding in public and expect to meet hostility. That's sad, because if breastfeeding is ever to become more accepted as 'normal,' then its profile needs to be raised."

For some women, like Brenda, although their confidence does grow as the baby grows, they never become completely happy breastfeeding "anywhere": *"At first I only breastfed in front of men if they were family members or new fathers. But as time went by, I learned to relax more in public. Before visiting cafes or art galleries, I would check to see if breastfeeding was permitted. I would use coatrooms or empty rooms whenever possible."*

Although there has been some increase in recent years in breastfeeding facilities in public places, there is still room for improvement. Some public facilities set a positive example by making it clear that breast-feeding is welcome.[47] Health Ministries in Canada advocate "Breastfeeding Anytime, Anywhere." There are no laws to restrict breastfeeding in public places in Canada. In the United States, laws have been passed in 10 states (Florida, Illinois, Iowa, Michigan, New York, Nevada, North Carolina, Texas, Utah and Virginia) protecting a mother's right to breastfeed in public. These laws clarify that breast-feeding is not indecent exposure, and thus not criminal behavior. Other states have similar bills pending.

To encourage and support women to be able to breastfeed for as long as they wish, there needs to be a wider awareness of the value of the breastfeeding relationship. More facilities are also needed in public places for women who choose to breastfeed privately.

Breastfeeding and Sex

The public confusion of breasts for breastfeeding and breasts as sex objects may spill over into your personal relationship with your part-ner. The relationship you may have taken for granted might have to be rethought. Many new parents wonder if breastfeeding will interfere with sex.

Giving birth is an intensely physical and emotional experience. Caring for a new baby is often all-engrossing. In so many ways, being preg-nant, giving birth and caring for a new baby disrupts your sexual rela-tionship as a couple. No matter how many books you read or classes you attend, you cannot ever truly prepare for the changes that a baby brings. During this time you need to maintain your sexual relationship as a couple according to constantly changing circumstances.

It may not be openly discussed in our society, but some men find their partners quite sexy when they are breastfeeding. This could be a result of the increase in breast size. Or it may be some more deep-seated emotional satisfaction.

Lynn describes how her sexual relationship with her husband deep-ened: *"My husband found my breasts very sexy after the birth of our daughter—particularly my nipples. He found they were larger (or more prominent). Nursing had softened them, drawing them out. I also found*

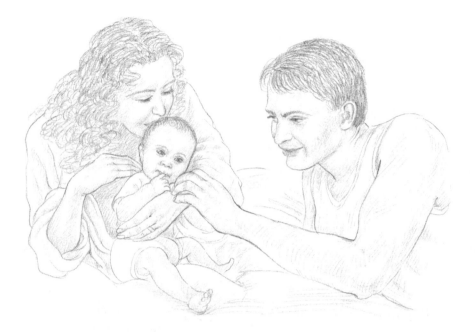

my nipples more sensitive and enjoyed them being touched when we made love—far more than before. I'd also lost some of my inhibitions about having my breasts touched during sex. I'd become more 'at home' with my body while breastfeeding. Leaking milk became a joke rather than a problem and we were happy to put a towel under my breasts. I feel sharing the birth experience together and having my husband's support during breastfeeding helped me enjoy and share my body more with him when we made love. Tiredness and sleepless nights were far worse for our sexual relationship than breastfeeding!"

Some women, such as Sharon, are aware of a great change resulting from their experience of birth and mothering. This can bring new confidence: *"Before I breastfed, I was self-conscious about my breasts, my figure and weight. I was absorbed in being a successful career woman who was as close to perfect as possible. Now, after breastfeeding, I feel so womanly and OK with my weight and figure (even though I'm still 20 pounds overweight). I feel confident in a way I never knew existed!"*

In the early months of a baby's life, you may both be exhausted physically and emotionally. You may find it hard to get enough sleep. Your sex drive may be temporarily channeled into other activities. Once you have begun to make love again after the birth, you may have other kinds of problems to deal with together, as Colette relates: *"I frequently felt so engorged I couldn't stand my husband touching me. I also found out later on (baby about seven months) that breastfeeding inhibits vaginal secretions for some women, presumably because it inhibits ovulation and production of estrogen. For me, it made intercourse very sore and painful. Until I learned this, I was worried about what could be wrong with me. I had visions of having been stitched up too tightly after birth or something. I wish the doctor had told me about this."*

The hormone that prompts milk let-down from the breasts—oxytocin—is the hormone involved in orgasm. You might breastfeed your baby before making love to keep from being showered by milk.

Or do as Linda did: *"Sex was more fulfilling after birth for both of us, though my husband kept clear of my breasts until about 12 months after the birth. Although I was still breastfeeding, that was when my breasts stopped leaking. Wearing a bra with pads in helped prevent interruptions because milk was leaking during breast stimulation by my husband."*

If you both can share your positive and negative feelings, your relationship is far more likely to remain healthy and emotionally nourishing for you. Sadly, sometimes the arrival of a baby brings real problems in a relationship to the surface. At such times expert help from a counselor can help many couples talk through their concerns together.

Most couples are able to work together to ensure their sexual relationship continues. You may even explore new areas of stimulation and enjoyment together at this time.

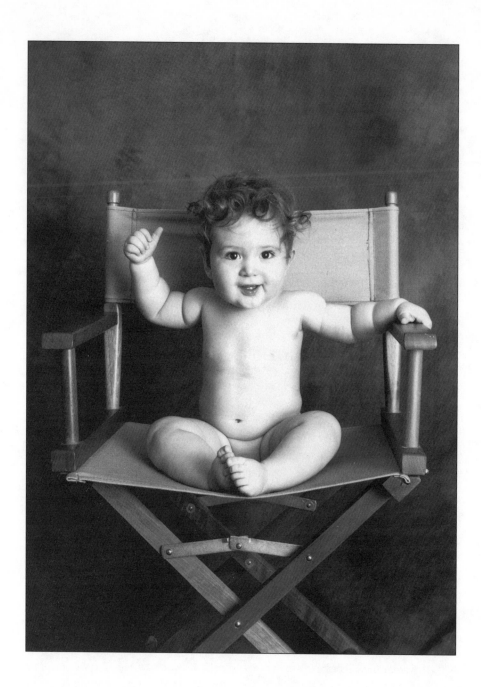

CHAPTER 6 *Moving Towards Independence*

When your baby is about six months old (younger in some babies, older in others), you will begin to introduce food other than breast milk to him. It is a new experience for him. It represents a movement away from the secure, natural and comforting activity of being cradled in his mother's arms while nursing.

Introducing Other Food

Introducing other foods ends your baby's total dependence on you. Women react in different ways to this event. Some are pleased. Others are sad to see their baby taking his first moves away from them. Some second-time mothers may delay introducing other foods because they don't want the baby to grow up too soon or cope with the extra chores involved. Your baby's first reactions may not be too positive. Instead of the pleasure of a soft, warm breast, your baby must get used to the feel of a hard, possibly cold spoon, first touching his lips and then being placed in his mouth. Go gently and gradually. There is no rush. Breast milk will remain the most valuable food for him for quite some time.

Irene began her baby on solids slowly at about 4½ months. There were no major problems: *"Life seems to get better and better. By the time she was eating three meals a day, she was still nursing from the breast six to eight times a day. This slowly dwindled to four to six times a day by the time she was a year old, and later to three to four times a day."*

It was similar for Sandy and her baby: *"I started to wean Linda at about five months. It was a gradual process. She took solids well. As she had more solids, she gradually cut out breastfeedings. It seemed to be a very natural process that she dictated. By her first birthday, Linda was having one breastfeeding when she woke up and one before bed."*

Your new baby cannot digest complex foods. Health Canada and the U.S. Department of Health and Human Services recommend exclusive breastfeeding for at least the first four to six months. So do the American Academy of Pediatrics, American Dietetic Associacian, Canadian Paediatric Society and the Canadian Dietetic Association. These groups encourage breastfeeding into the second year of life, with the gradual introduction of solids to meet the needs of the growing child. To prevent allergies, it is better to wait until about six months, if possible, before introducing solids. A baby's capacity to digest and use other foods is determined by the maturity of his stomach—his age—not by his weight or the length of time he sleeps.

As his digestion matures, new enzymes are produced that help him digest other foods as well as milk. However, during the first two years of life, breast milk is the easiest source of food for your baby. He will continue to derive a high nutritional benefit from breast milk. Starting other foods can be as low-key as possible. The idea is to offer the baby a chance to try new tastes and textures. Many mothers begin with baby cereal mixed with breast milk. The familiar smell of your breast milk may comfort your baby. Introduce one new taste at a time. This way, your baby's reaction to each one can be watched, particularly if there is a history of food allergies in the family.

"I was still nursing frequently at night so this time (a second baby) I introduced solids, hoping she might sleep longer. She loved the solids, but it didn't make a difference as far as the number of breastfeedings she had."

This was Debbie's experience. Like many mothers, she had heard that starting solid food helps a baby sleep longer at night. Or that it may reduce the number of times he nurses at night. If you think about the amounts involved in the early stages of weaning, this idea seems unlikely. Since a baby cannot fully digest more complex foods until he is older, the amount of breast milk he receives remains important. Sometimes a baby may even wake more often to get the milk he needs, like Joe, Dawn's baby, did: *"When Joe was about nine weeks old, he became difficult to satisfy. By this time he weighed 15 pounds. I suggested to my pediatrician that I start to introduce solids. I knew that this was earlier than the accepted three to four months. But Joe was much heavier than expected for babies of his age.*

"To begin with, I was very careful of what I gave Joe. He started with baby rice, mixed with expressed breast milk. Then I followed with various puréed fruits and vegetables. Pretty soon he showed a liking for stronger flavors. By the time he was 6 months, he was eating breakfast, lunch and dinner. He was still nursing from me first thing in the morning, mid-morning, mid-afternoon and at bedtime. But then he slept through the night until morning."

A young baby connects the satisfaction of easing hunger with sucking. When he cries from hunger, he expects to suck. In the early stages of weaning, it may be useful to breastfeed first and then offer a taste of

FEEDING FILE

Tips for introducing other foods

- Try not to be influenced too much by what other babies are doing, or their eating or sleeping patterns.
- If your baby is younger than four months, try increasing the breast milk he receives before starting other foods.
- Offer his first tastes *after* nursing him.
- Sometime after starting solids your baby may accept a "breast sandwich"; that is, one breast, then solids, then the other breast.
- Start at a relaxed time of the day.
- Hold the baby on your knee for the first tastes.
- Use a flat, small, sturdy plastic spoon. Place it on the baby's lips and let him "lap" his first tastes.
- Simple puréed fruits may be easy starter foods.
- If he doesn't like it, leave it a few days and try again.

- Use prepared baby food if it is easier for you. This keeps you from feeling he is rejecting your own prepared food.
- Read the labels, so you know what he is getting.
- If he has had enough, let him tell you. Don't force it.
- Offer a fairly wide selection of tastes. He may like what you do not.
- If he is not feeling well, he may not accept other foods. Go back to fully breastfeeding until he feels better.
- Breast milk is a good base for a mixed diet. As long as your baby is taking plenty of breast milk, you can wean to solids at a leisurely pace.
- Contact a La Leche League leader, a lactation consultant, or WIC staff (Women, Infants and Children nutritional program for women with low incomes in the United States) for weaning tips.

the new food. Hold your baby in your arms to reassure him. Use a fairly flat, sturdy plastic spoon to help things go smoothly. Make the first foods very "runny." Your baby can "lap" from a flat spoon when it is placed to his lips. Good, gentle experiences for your baby will set the scene for later feedings. As time passes, your baby will accept greater amounts of food and a wide range of tastes and textures.

When Elaine's baby, David, was three months old, she introduced solids in the form of baby cereal mixed with some of her expressed breast milk: *"I also gave him gluten-free, low-sugar baby toast, which I softened with a little boiled water. Then I added a little of my expressed milk to give him the familiar taste and smell. He would eat this right away, and sometimes wanted more! I would follow with a breastfeeding. He took to solids well. By four months he was having breakfast, lunch and dinner, followed by a breastfeeding."*

Some women do not find it easy to introduce other foods to their baby. There is no doubt that new foods mean there will be more washing-up, more messy clothes and smellier diapers to deal with. There is also the decision about what to feed a baby at this stage. Labels on food products such as "sugar-free," "gluten-free," "best for baby," "fortified with" or "additional factor X" all seem to confuse parents. A multi-million-dollar industry produces and markets baby foods. Slick ads could make you believe that your baby needs a certain food—or, worse, that the product is somehow better than what you can produce simply and easily in your kitchen. That's not true. What *is* true is, baby-food companies don't make money if you buy a fresh banana and mash it for your baby!

If your baby does not like a taste, he may close his mouth or let the food dribble out of his mouth. If you have spent some time fixing a special food for your baby, it might be hard to accept his reaction. You might feel a bit rejected. You may be tempted to continue offering the food. (Ready-made foods have a psychological advantage here. It is much easier to throw away food that has come from a box!) These natural responses come from connecting food with love.

Try to be aware of your feelings. Don't let your emotions become too involved with the food you are making. Some women stick with exclusive breastfeeding until their babies are ready to start solids—and they themselves are ready to make that effort. No need to hurry. There is evidence that exclusive breastfeeding for at least the first 13 weeks will benefit your baby's health.[48]

Breastfeeding the Older Baby

Breastfeeding an older baby is a special experience. Each baby has a unique personality and there is a lot to enjoy together, as Patti describes: *"A high point I will always remember was when my 14-month-old daughter sucked twice to get the let down started. Then she looked up at me, grinned, then disappeared below my blouse, where she blew a 'raspberry' on my tummy as a joke. Of course she was latched on in time to catch the rush of milk."*

For Lesley, the pleasure of breastfeeding has increased with time: *"Eleven months later, the milk is still on tap. We both enjoy the closeness and comfort that nursing gives. I keep meaning to cut down Mary's feedings to two a day—first thing in the morning and last thing at night. But we can't cut down on the cuddles and 'snacks' in between. Well, there's not much of problem with that. Breastfeeding won't last forever. And really we're both making the most of it while we can. What's wrong with that?"*

Choosing to continue breastfeeding may mean that you will be exposed to comments and criticism. The attitudes of others are not always supportive. There seems to be an unwritten law: breastfeeding is all right, but not in public or when the baby is older. The question then is what constitutes an "older baby." There may be as many suggestions as there are people willing to voice them! Common ideas are: not when the baby can eat other food, not once he has teeth, not when she can wear shoes and walk.

Some families seem to raise the issue that breastfeeding a baby beyond a certain age could lead to something sexual. Often, sexual matters are not discussed openly in families. In such cases disapproval might be expressed only indirectly. The following explanations have been offered to some women: Breastfeeding a boy child too long could mean that he becomes too attached to his mother, or develops too great an interest in women's breasts as an adult, while breastfeeding a girl child beyond a certain age may reduce her capacity to relate well to men. There is no evidence for any of these tales.

Vanessa describes how amazed she was when she came across this type of prejudice in her own family: *"One of my father's cousins breastfed her little boy until he was about four. I remember family rumblings about it.*

Looking back, I think two factors influenced their thinking. First, that she was somehow 'spoiling' the boy, indulging him. By 'allowing' him to continue to have access to her whenever he liked, they felt she was not asserting her own will. Second, there was a concern regarding sexuality. It was felt that she might be deriving some sensual pleasure from this form of contact. Nature has designed the breastfeeding species. Why deny its sensuality? It seems that there is often more concern when the child still breastfeeding is a boy!"

Sometimes objections are also raised that breastfeeding can harm your physical health, or that you will become too dependent upon your child for emotional satisfaction. Again, there is no evidence to support this.

Hearing these kinds of comments or just being aware that something is disapproved of can lead to a lot of soul-searching. Sometimes you may begin to feel you have to defend what you are doing. You may have to be assertive or develop a "tough" layer, as Amy discovered with her third baby when he was 18 months old: *"The other day someone asked me, 'What is it like to nurse a toddler who is walking?' All I could think to say was that it wasn't strange, and then I found myself saying, 'Well, it isn't like nursing a toddler. I am nursing Robert, just like I have since he was born.' When I thought about this incident later, my reply reminded me of the ongoing nature of the nursing relationship. It is very much a two-way thing, not strictly under your control because it involves another person. With my third child, I had no preconceived ideas about when I might wean him. I was ready to trust my own instincts rather than seeking outside opinions."*

Sunita also experienced critical comments: *"Outside the home, I was very aware of embarrassment while nursing a toddler. Even before she was a year old, people would remark on her still being 'attached.' I also ran into some hostility when I took her to a local toddler-aerobics session. Feeling a little cranky, Jane asked to nurse. Once attached, I was informed that no food or drink was allowed. I really cannot view breastfeeding as being like other forms of food. I stalked off, feeling humiliated and embarrassed."*

You may not make a definite decision to continue breastfeeding. But if everything is comfortable between you and your baby, breastfeeding just becomes part of the day-to-day life you share. Breastfeeding may become a very small part of your life. The focus for other people may be different.

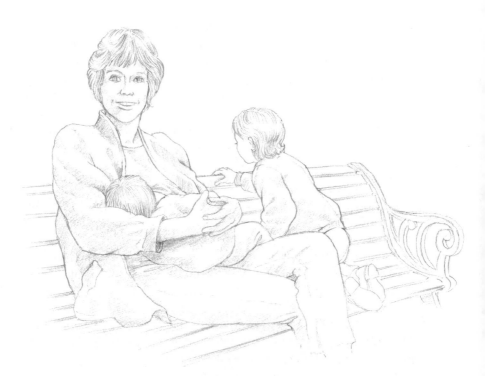

Irene nursed her baby for more than 19 months, but found the social pressures were getting stronger: *"I found the situation hard to cope with. I didn't think I was flaunting it. She rarely nursed unless we were at home (except if we were at a friend's at nap time). She didn't ask for it when we were out. And I felt good about it, despite some pretty strong comments. People I spoke to said things like: What was I doing still nursing at 19 months? Wasn't there a harmful effect on me? The people who did support 'longer' breastfeeding were wonderful. They made me feel much better about the 'Should I?' and 'Why?' questions. But I found most people were terribly insensitive."*

Sunita firmly believes that breastfeeding becomes more useful as your baby grows older: *"To me, it seemed natural to keep on doing what worked so well. What else calms an emotional toddler so easily and sends her off to sleep in a matter of minutes? Toddlers rarely understand their own emotions and can't really cope with them. Neither can we as adults cope with our toddlers at times. Breastfeeding calms both them and us so well."*

Some women decide to deal with negative comments by gaining more information. They make a very positive choice to keep breastfeeding their babies. Others, like Paula, acknowledge the benefits of longer breastfeeding. They appreciate the closeness that breastfeeding provides in all sorts of situations: *"As I write this, Charlotte is 14 months old. I don't feel an urge to be done with breastfeeding. I believe that breast milk continues to be important during the second year of life. There are times—for example, when she may be slightly ill—that she will refuse solid foods. I can offer her my breast, which is a great comfort to her. Breast milk is easily digested and nourishing for a feverish baby, too. I feel a special closeness to her when she is feeling bad, and I am thankful that I can respond to her in such an intimate, physical way.*

"On a more day-to-day level, Charlotte has turned out to be a fussy eater. Her diet consists largely of peanut-butter sandwiches and garlic bread. She refuses all fruit and vegetables (except potatoes and corn). Breast milk is an important part of her limited diet. In fact, it is probably her only decent source of nutrition!

"I think that breast milk is a solid back-up against the uncertainties of ill health and poor eating. It is kind of like my insurance policy. For me, breastfeeding creates a perfect way to respond to my baby with passion, tenderness, comfort and, of course, love."

Vanessa and her partner both acknowledge the special bond of breastfeeding: *"I am now aware that there are physical benefits in breastfeeding the older baby. (Rachel will soon be two.) I am still passing antibodies to her through my milk. I also believe that the emotional benefits, to both of us, are enormous. She can find comfort from my breast. And I am able to give comfort in a unique and loving way.*

"I particularly enjoy nursing before bedtime. It is a quiet, private and peaceful time for both of us. I love the fact that she can not only communicate her desire for 'mommy milk' but she can express her enjoyment of it. In reply to my asking if it's nice, she nods her head vigorously. Although breastfeeding gives Rachel and me a special relationship, it is quite an exclusive one. My husband and I have had to acknowledge that and talk about this. At times it has meant totally separate bedtime routines for us and our children. Without his understanding and support, it would have been difficult to continue breastfeeding.

"I'm pleased my breastfeeding journey with Rachel has gone so well, particularly because she is a girl. It seems important to me. I suppose it's because I hope that one day she will be able to experience for herself those same feelings of joy that I felt while nursing her. I must admit to

being a 'closet' breastfeeder now. While Rachel was still a baby, that is, crawling and gurgling, I was at ease breastfeeding in public. Now I feel less inclined. For one thing, I have gone back to wearing normal, underwire bras. They make access to my breasts less easy. And it is harder to be discreet when nursing a toddler. Rachel tends to pull my clothing and wants to play with my other nipple while nursing. I still do not feel ready to give up this precious, privileged, mutually enjoyable process. I know it will be over one day. I suppose it will happen gradually. And maybe I won't realize that the last breastfeeding has happened."

Nursing a toddler can be funny at times, as Julie, mother of 3-year-old Penny, describes: *"There is a social joy in feeding an older child you don't get with a baby. Every morning we walked with Sara, my older daughter, to her nursery school. And when we got home Penny would say, 'Shall we have a nice drink, Mommy?' She often commented if it was a particularly nice taste. And once she guessed correctly that I had eaten some pineapples! One day she said that it was so nice today that she'd try the other side. Would it be the same?*

"I never suffered the problems that many women describe when nursing older children who 'demand' it at inconvenient times. Or use words mother finds embarrassing at the supermarket checkout. Between us we sorted out without discussing it that Penny had her 'nice drink' at certain times when we could both sit down and enjoy it. She only used to breastfeed for comfort when she was ill."

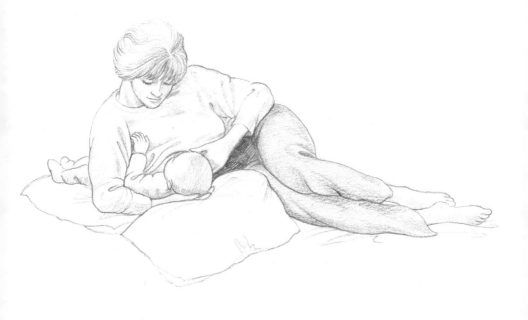

Breastfeeding can be very useful during times of illness, as Joy found with her baby Maggie: *"My youngest daughter Maggie was breastfed until just before her third birthday. She stopped when she decided she didn't need to nurse at night. At about 18 months, Maggie had a horrible bout of chickenpox. She was covered with spots, even her mouth. The back of her throat was swollen and spotty. She refused to put a cup to her mouth because it was too sore. I was relieved to be able to fully breastfeed her for a few days. Like her sisters, she tends to get wheezy colds. Letting her nurse at night when she could have longer, comfort sucking, worked much better, and was less exhausting for both of us, than spending the night in a steamy bathroom."*

Leigh knows that her daughter Emily relishes her "mommy milk." For her too it has been a time of great self-awareness: *"I've enjoyed the closeness it brought us as Emily developed from baby to preschool child. It has been a handy soother and the ultimate fast-food snack. Stopping slowly is giving each of us a chance to find other ways of being close and expressing our love. I feel a tremendous bond with my daughter. This is in part because of our long breastfeeding relationship."*

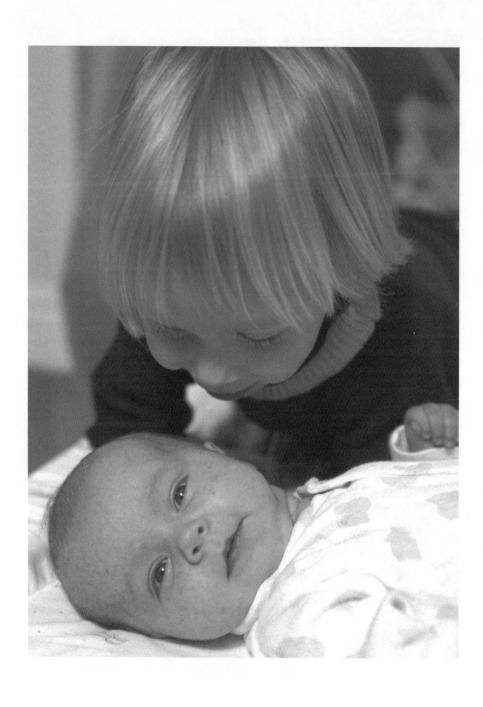

CHAPTER 7 ## *A Breastfeeding Family*

Another Baby?

It may be an effort for you as a mother of one child to take the time to prepare your body and mind for the next birth. Attending prenatal classes may not be easy when you have other children to care for. If you do arrange care for your older child and attend prenatal classes or a refresher course, you will find it is a real pleasure to focus on yourself and the new baby. Making time to think about what it will be like to have another baby to care for is all-important. Focus on both day-to-day and emotional concerns. It is just as important to take time to enjoy thinking about your coming baby!

Practical concerns include: "Where will the new baby sleep?," "How will we all fit in the car?," "What will happen to the toddler while I'm in labor?," "Will there be enough money coming in?"

Emotional concerns often center on worries about coping with the demands of the first child while handling the demands of a new baby: "Can there be enough hours in the day?," "How will it feel to relate to two or maybe three little children?," "Who do we feed first?," "How will the older child behave?," "Whose needs come first?" There are so many questions to consider.

Perhaps the underlying question is: "How can it be possible to love another child as much as I love this one?" Even if there has been a difficult start with the first baby and the path of parenthood has been bumpy, most men and women fall hopelessly in love with their children. There is nothing more wonderful for a parent than to have a small, trusting hand clutched in yours or to feel the unconditional love we might

---

FEEDING FILE

Thinking about Another Baby and Breastfeeding

Before the baby arrives

- Try to spend time talking with your older child about the arrival of another baby.
- Photographs of him as a baby will show him how helpless he once was.
- Photographs of him nursing or meeting other breastfed babies would help him learn about breastfeeding.
- Do not expect him to share your joy at the prospect of another baby. And don't tell him how lucky he will be to have a playmate. New babies are not good at playing anything!
- If your toddler still has a daytime nap, try to preserve it. That short quiet time during the afternoon will be really helpful for you after the baby arrives.
- It might be possible to get a doll and cradle for your older child. He could care for "his" baby while you care for the new one.
- If possible, do not plan major changes near the time of the birth of the new baby. It is enough to get used to having a new baby brother or sister without starting preschool, too, for example.

- There may be picture books at the library showing home life that could lead to talks about what life with a new baby might be like. For example: "Sometimes Daddy will get breakfast. Mommy will have to nurse a lot."
- If your toddler is of that age, put off potty training until well after the new baby comes.
- Get him to sit with you as you rest towards the end of your pregnancy. There will be times when you are nursing the new baby when your older child can sit with you as you nurse. When you are breastfeeding, you will have an arm free to cuddle him.
- Choose a box of toys that will only be brought out when you're breastfeeding. Let your toddler choose which toys go in that box. Maybe give it a special name, so that he knows both the box of toys and breastfeeding are special.

---

receive from our children. These are truly very special moments. Some of this "reward" explains why many couples choose to have more than one child.

Some planning ahead about coping with two (or more) children is useful, but much of the future as a family is really wait-and-see. It helps to know that most parents find the "amount" of love available grows with each additional child. It is not a case of having to divide the "amount" of love by the number of children.

FEEDING FILE

Thinking about Another Baby and Breastfeeding

After the baby is born

- The new baby competes for your attention. Moving your toddler from being the baby to the "big boy" in the family is quite a challenge. Be prepared to be patient.

- Try to think ahead and have a drink, a snack, a book or toys ready for your older child before you start to breastfeed the new baby.

- It is worthwhile to spend time with your older child when the new baby sleeps. Resist the urge to dash around doing chores. Your older child is your baby, too. He will need a lot of reassurance that you still love him. Spending time with him is the best assurance you can offer.

- Your older child may ask to try out your breast milk. He may even remember nursing himself. Try to accept his request. Go through the motions of giving him your breast. He may not remember how to nurse and will likely lose interest. Those youngsters who can nurse often don't like the taste of breast milk. Entertaining his natural curiosity helps his interest pass to something else.

- Talk to your older child. Tell him how you feel. Ask him how *he* feels. He will understand much more than you might think. He may even pick up on your tensions. By talking, you may be able to stay more relaxed. It is worth a try.

- Life will be pretty hectic as you adjust to caring for more than one child. But it does get easier.

- Your older child does not need a busy social life at this time. He needs you in a good state of mind much more. Invest in plenty of home activities for the older child, such as play-clay, paper and glue, construction toys. Cut out all but essential trips. Conserve your energies, just for the time being.

- Get help from relatives and friends who are familiar to your child. A short time spent away from you and the new baby may ease any tension that develops.

- Some churches or community centers organize parent, baby and toddler groups.

- La Leche League groups often organize days when you can nurse with other mothers while the older children play together. Visiting with other mothers always helps.

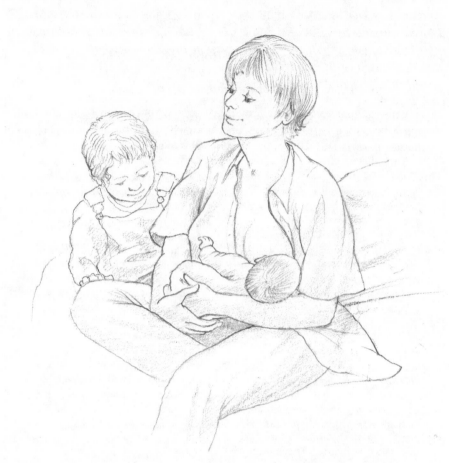

Tandem Nursing

Quite a few women stop breastfeeding to help their menstrual cycle return to normal so they may conceive another baby. It is also possible to become pregnant while you are still breastfeeding your baby or toddler. Some older babies naturally "go off" breast milk at this point. The taste may change because of the changing hormones in your bloodstream. Your nipples may become quite sensitive during the early stages of pregnancy. You may consciously or unconsciously encourage your baby or toddler to stop breastfeeding.

Anna nursed her first baby until she was three: *"She loved nursing and I loved nursing her. Gradually she nursed less, as other things became important to her. She stopped when I became pregnant. Perhaps the milk tasted different or there wasn't as much of it. She wasn't upset about it. She just didn't want to nurse any more."*

If the early stages of your next pregnancy pass without your older child stopping breastfeeding, you may find yourself thinking about breastfeeding both the new baby and your toddler—tandem nursing.

This may not always be easy to do, as Dawn explains: *"I breastfed my first child for two years and three months. In fact, I was still nursing her while in labor with my son. Once nursing was established, my son was voracious and doubled his birth weight at nine weeks. I tried to nurse both children, but my supply just matched my toddler's demands. I quickly became exhausted. My healthcare provider said I had to stop nursing my toddler right away. She explained to my daughter why she couldn't have 'milkies' any more. I now know that I should have made greater efforts before the baby's birth to wean her. The whole episode was very painful and traumatic for both of us."*

Dawn had a mixed experience. While she kept breastfeeding during pregnancy, she seemed to be responding to the needs of her toddler. But once the baby was born things became more complex.

Laurie found that she really enjoyed tandem feeding: *"My oldest child, nearly three, was still nursing when her sister was born. It was a really special feeling to have both of my children cuddled up to me, nursing together. Before her sister was born, the eldest was only nursing three or four times a day. But for the first month or so afterwards, she wanted to nurse every time the baby did. That made it a lot easier for me: no trying to amuse a bored and jealous toddler while breastfeeding the new baby. We just sat and relaxed together. I was confident that my body would respond to the extra suckling, and it did. I had tons of milk, so never had to worry about whether the baby would get enough."*

If you are in this situation, it helps to allow your new baby free and first access to your breasts in the early weeks. This ensures that the new baby receives the vital colostrum and has a chance to build up his own milk supply.

Worries

For some women, a second pregnancy may bring very real worries about nursing; Sophie explains: *"Pregnant,' I heard myself saying, 'How wonderful!' A baby brother or sister for my 5-year-old son, Paul. The excitement of the news wore off when I remembered the horrible time I had breastfeeding Paul. I spent the first six weeks of my son's life trying to force my breasts upon him! The pain, the tears and the frustration! Well, not this time—I was in control with this baby. I'd already been there, done that and failed. What was the point of putting me and my new baby through all that, when I knew perfectly well that breastfeeding was not for me? No, the decision had been made, no breastfeeding this baby—bottles here we come! Having made the decision, I sat back and enjoyed the next nine months. Everything was clear in my head about my preferred method of feeding."*

Martha expects her second baby soon and plans to bottle-feed from the start: *"Although I understand that there were many reasons why I rejected my daughter, I am convinced that breastfeeding played a major part in my depression. I am equally certain that things will be better this time, now the burden of guilt of not breastfeeding has been lifted."*

Rebecca is pregnant again: *"This time I have an open mind. If breastfeeding works, well then, I will breastfeed. If it doesn't, I will bottle-feed. I would like to know what it is like to nurse a baby. I would like to give my baby the best food possible. And I would like to avoid the expense and hassle of buying and fixing formula. But if breastfeeding doesn't work out, I know bottle-feeding is not the end of the world."*

Often, second and subsequent births are easier, and breastfeeding can begin in a relaxed and gentle way. The 1990 Infant Feeding Survey[1] found women were more likely to breastfeed the second baby if they had breastfed the first.

This was certainly the case for Vanessa: *"With Rachel, my second baby, the birth was so different. She was born into water in a quiet and dimly lit room. She was put to my breast within the first hour of her life and nursed for a little while. She slept a lot that day but woke towards the evening and had her first 'real' feeding. I felt confident enough to try nursing her lying down in the hospital bed (something I never mastered the first time). The hospital staff left me alone—they could see I was fine."*

Tanya also found the second time around easier: *"I had no real prob-lems when my second child was born at home 11 months ago. I was still anxious the first few days, waiting for my milk supply to establish itself."*

Carly had a bad breastfeeding experience the first time: *"But this time it was different. My baby settled down and she slept. I believed in myself. I knew this time what I had to offer was the very best. No one could dif-fuse my nurturing instinct."*

If you have had a difficult breastfeeding experience with your first baby, you may need to come to terms with a lot of mixed feelings. There may be a sense of your body letting you down in some way. You may wonder why breastfeeding was so hard when it is supposed to be a natural process. You might also wonder if it is worth trying again. There could be the chance that it will not go well and so there could be further disappointment.

Some women cope with these feelings of disappointment at the time, crying and expressing their feelings to those around them. Gradually they may be able to put the experience behind them. But some women will have dealt with their disappointment by burying it, not talking about it or discussing it. If you are in this situation, it is possible that the fears you have about breastfeeding will surface as the expected date of delivery of the next baby draws near. In this case, it is really important that you try to talk through your worries. Speak with your doctor or midwife, a lactation consultant, or a La Leche League leader.

It does take courage to try again. Many women have their courage rewarded the second or third time around, like Lorna: *"One baby girl born in July, 1994, safe and sound. 'Bring in the bottles,' I heard myself say. My husband wanted me to at least try to breastfeed. So reluctantly I tried to latch Kyra on to my breast. I was thinking that I'll show him, I'll try it, fail miserably like last time and he'll feel guilty and let me bottle-feed after all. Wrong! Kyra latched on to my breast and nursed away happily. It's been that way ever since—no engorgement, no cracked nipples, no pain. Just one very happy baby. I still can't believe it, six months later. I hated breastfeeding the first time. It was the worst time of my life. But with my second baby, I have loved every minute of it. I'm so glad that my husband encouraged me to try again. I wouldn't have missed breastfeeding my daughter for the world."*

Sandra kept trying: *"It has taken me three attempts and three babies to achieve successful breastfeeding. Now having nursed Joel for six months. I know there will be no bottles for him. No, this time breast is best. I am proud to have overcome my problems."*

Gail defied her family's skepticism. With the birth of her third child, she decided to try breastfeeding once more: *"This time, I decided to ask for help from anyone who could. I met a lactation consultant during my pregnancy and told her about my previous problems and how I still wanted to overcome them. By the time I got home with Nathan (day four), I was fairly confident. I was soon hitching up my T-shirt whenever he opened his mouth. As a successful breastfeeder (at last) there is a wonderful feeling of fulfillment. Best of all, our two girls get to see their mother breastfeed. I hope they will remember that in the future."*

Of course, breastfeeding a second or third child means that there is a toddler or older child to care for as well. Many women meet together, sometimes in each other's homes, during the early days with a second

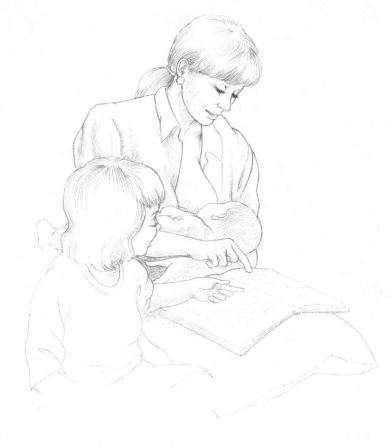

or subsequent baby. The older children have company while their mothers talk and offer each other support. Also, by breastfeeding, at least there will be one arm and hand free to give affection to the other child, as Jinny and Laura discovered: *"I loved the ease, especially because I now had a toddler I was trying to keep track of as well. It became our special quiet time. I would nurse and Jacob would curl up on the other side with a book or a puzzle. We would read or sing songs to the baby. And having a toddler, breastfeeding was my time to really concentrate on the baby, with eye-to-eye and skin-to-skin contact. When my husband was home, he could entertain the toddler. I was much more active the second time. I had more errands to run, more places to be or to take Jacob. I found the ease of nursing really helped.*

"Some of my happiest memories of that time are sitting down in the cool of our family room—nursing the baby with my arm around his sister, reading her a story. I asked myself then, and I still do now, how could I have coped with holding a baby and feeding him while holding a book and turning the pages if I'd been bottle-feeding?"

Laurie found herself a source of entertainment: *"When my third daughter was born, the eldest was nearly six. She was able to understand when I breastfed the two younger children. Sometimes she joined me on the sofa and 'breastfed' her doll too!"*

Breastfeeding Twins or More

Some couples learn, during the pregnancy, that they are to be the parents of two babies. The dilemmas faced by parents of children that are born one at a time come all at once to the parents of twins or more. An instant family: double trouble or twice the pleasure? Learning that you are expecting twins—or more—may cause you to wonder if you can nurse them both yourself. Women often have little confidence that their bodies can produce enough milk for one baby. When there are two babies, many mothers believe that it will not be possible to fully breastfeed them both.

In the past, women have always been able to feed more than one baby. Wet nurses often took on four to six babies at once.[49] The laws of supply and demand still operate. If two babies are breastfeeding, your breasts will produce enough for two. A study in 1977 found that the prolactin response in women who are breastfeeding twins may be double that of mothers nursing only one baby.[50]

FEEDING FILE

Breastfeeding Twins or More

One at a time or both at once?

The first decision you will be faced with is "one at a time" or "both together". Perhaps nursing one baby at a time at first can help you overcome problems with that baby. It may help you get to know each of your babies. Nursing them together becomes easier as the babies get older and better at latching on. But nursing both together provides more stimulation to the milk supply. So this tactic may be useful to build up a good supply. If you have help, you may choose to nurse both together for this reason.

Positions for feeding

When it comes to bringing the babies together to your breasts, there are several ways to proceed.

The **"football hold"** is a good position for newborn twins. Place the babies so that their body and legs are tucked under your arms, and their heads and necks are supported in your hands. Hold the babies so that they are tucked in to your sides, with their tummies facing you. Use pillows to give extra support, so you are not bending over the babies. As the babies gain control of their heads, you will not need to support their heads. This leaves your arms free to hold a drink or read a book.

For the **"parallel hold,"** hold one of the babies in the "normal" nursing position (across your body). Hold the other in the "football" hold, so that the babies are lying parallel with each other, facing the same direction. Again, you'll need pillows to support the babies so you are not supporting any weight. Hold the babies so their tummies are facing you.

It is possible to hold both babies in the conventional nursing position, with one baby lying across the other. This is called the **"crisscross hold."**

It is important to check that both babies are in the correct position, with their bodies facing you. There are no special rules for positioning twins, just the normal rules for good positioning. Each mother will learn for herself which position works best. You will find your babies have their own preferences, too.

Choosing a breast

Some mothers choose to swap their babies to the other breast at each feeding. Others prefer to keep one breast for each baby.

Swapping breasts regularly helps you maintain an even supply. This is an advantage if one baby is stronger than the other. The stronger sucker will stimulate the supply for the weaker. But keeping each baby to his own breast may be better for establishing that baby's milk supply to suit him. It will ensure he gets enough hindmilk for growth. Some babies may prefer one breast. Again, this is something you will learn for yourself as your babies grow.

If you have already breastfed a baby, you are more likely to look forward to nursing more than one with optimism. You may find that other people—even your healthcare providers—are skeptical about your ability to breastfeed more than one baby. It helps if you are able to talk to someone who is already nursing twins. If you have supportive healthcare providers, you may anticipate rather than dread the experience.

> **Further help with twins or more**
>
> Call Twinline, in Berkeley, California, at (510) 524-0863.
>
> Twinline (Twin Services) provides useful written and recorded information for parents of twins or more.

For Donna, the reality was even more complex—three babies! *"After getting over the shock of expecting triplets, and staggering through the first few months of pregnancy, I got in touch with other triplet parents. It helped to discuss the 'realities' of a multiple birth. I discussed how to breastfeed triplets with several families. I had accepted that our babies would have to be breast- and bottle-fed if we were to survive. We had also accepted that our babies were likely to spend a few weeks in an intensive-care unit. Therefore I would need to use a breast pump so they could be tube/bottle-fed when I was not there."*

Olivia's first child was a delight to nurse: *"So when I found I was pregnant with twins two years later, I'd had a positive experience to convince me I definitely wanted to breastfeed again. But I had a lot of opposition from various people who feared that Brianna would somehow miss out, or I wouldn't have enough milk. La Leche League was great because I was lucky enough to have a leader in my area who had herself breastfed twins."*

Often a mother has to contend with the serious doubts of "the experts": *"All the medical staff were skeptical about breastfeeding twins. Thankfully I was in contact with other mothers of twins who had breastfed and enjoyed it. So I was determined to go ahead. I read everything positive about nursing twins and ignored the rest. I had to keep telling my doctor that I was not going to 'try' breastfeeding both, but that I was going to."*

An added problem for you as the mother of twins may be that your babies are born early. Prematurity is common with twin births. This may complicate getting breastfeeding started. If the babies are too small to nurse, you will need to express your milk until they can go to the breast.

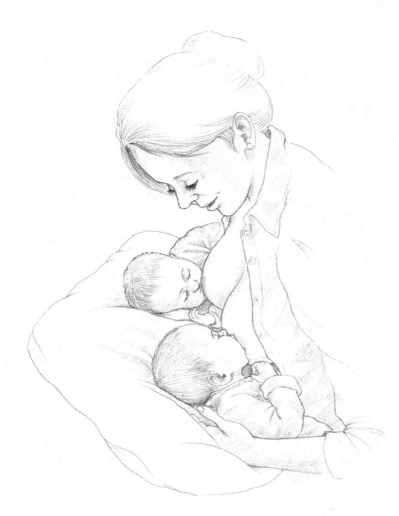

It is important that your doctor understands your desire to breastfeed and gives positive help and encouragement from the start. Sometimes, if the babies are near term, the birth may be really tiring. Thoughts of putting babies to your breasts may be the last thing on your mind.

It certainly was for Donna: *"The birth of our babies was a very exciting and wonderful event. It was also rather shocking—the doctor produced a fourth baby on delivery! My first words on receiving a fourth healthy baby cannot be repeated. They are only made acceptable because of the colorful language of the three, not four, pediatricians present at the birth.*

"I began to express breast milk about 30 hours after delivery. That was the earliest I could possibly have tried to do anything other than sleep. I burst into tears."

Helpful and supportive caregivers are essential in the early days, says Pat: *"It wasn't until I was moved to a room as a postnatal mother that I tried to give the twins their first feeding. The night-shift nurses had just come on. I was lucky to be assigned a really helpful and supportive nurse. She found some cushions and a V-shaped pillow, which I placed across my lap. This helped me support the babies, so I could nurse them both at once."*

In common with other mothers, mothers of twins need good support and encouragement in the early weeks of breastfeeding. You will also need good practical help during the learning phase. Positioning two babies together may seem impossible to begin with.

Getting breastfeeding started with twins (or more) may seem like an impossible task. It may not be made easy by those around you, as Hilary remembers vividly: *"I insisted on being helped to nurse each twin right after birth and again later. I knew that although breastfeeding was encouraged, the staff really didn't care. Ready-made bottles were offered all the time. They told me I'd have to supplement with bottles. I asked them to just let me handle it. I started nursing one baby at a time. I kept one breast for each so that my supply would adjust to the needs of each. I kept one twin on each side of the bed. When he was there, my partner would walk up and down with one baby while I'd nurse the other, then swap. But the waiting baby would scream all the time and this was hell. Many a nurse came to the door with a bottle of formula. We told them to please go away.*

"When my partner had not been there for a few hours, my spirits would drop. They insisted on feeding soya milk through a nasal tube. I would not let them give a bottle. The babies were sick and pulled the tubes out. So I decided to try nursing them both at the same time. A friend with twins had lent me a V-shaped pillow to put across my front to rest them on. This was the single most useful thing. It made keeping both babies in the right place much easier. (I recommend it for all nursing twins!) Until we got the hang of it, keeping both latched on was hard. But the peace when we did was bliss. And the sensation of both of them nursing was wonderful. There were no dripping breasts, either. And it went faster, too.

"After that, I stuck to this in the daytime. I'd call a nurse to hold one while I got the second latched on. By this time, the staff realized I was going to manage somehow. They were more helpful and quite impressed."

At first Pat found it hard to relax: *"Both babies seemed to be balanced on the pillow. I had only one pair of hands but two newborns. I found the nighttimes difficult during the first few days. I seemed to be up and down all night long, nursing one or the other of the twins. Some of the nurses were unsupportive, even critical. One nurse, herself the mother of twins, kept telling me to 'get them on the bottle.' I felt very upset and alone. All the other women nearby had one baby. And all were bottle-fed. I felt I was being stubborn."*

Once your babies are home, learning to cope can take some time. Mothers of twins quickly learn to accept all offers of help. They discover their own ways to get by. Should I nurse the babies together or one at a time?

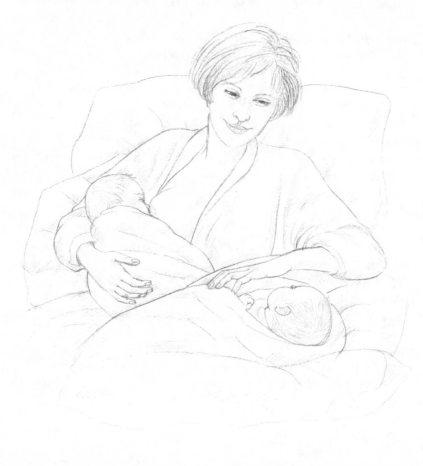

How do I pick up and hold two small babies? And how can I cope with a lively toddler as well? These are all common problems for a mother of twins.

Pat spent seven days in the hospital. Within that time her milk supply became established and bountiful. Both twins settled into a four-hour schedule: *"I never did get the hang of nursing two at once. One of the twins always nursed a little less and always threw up a few mouthfuls afterwards. Once I was at home, I learned to nurse whoever woke up first. I always offered my fullest breast. In the meantime, the other baby was placed in a little rocker which I gently moved with my foot. When the first baby finished nursing, he swapped places with his twin and the second baby got my second breast."*

Once Olivia's twins were home she tried different positions. She decided to nurse her babies one at a time: *"The main trouble I found when nursing them together was that I had a tremendous drop in blood sugar. My speech would slur and I felt faint. I had to sit with milk and a sandwich for me! I did feel very proud that I was able to satisfy two babies. However, Brianna and Courtney clearly had different appetites. It was hard to burp one baby while nursing the other. Also, I had decided to give the babies one breast each (Courtney on the left and Brianna on the right)! This meant that Brianna had the most 'difficult' nipple. When I'd tried to swap them around, I became confused. I worried about one baby getting too much or too little hindmilk. So I began nursing them one at a time. I felt it was a special way to relate with each child."*

Meg learned that it was easier for her to nurse both twins together: *"I was finally allowed to bring the twins home at six days old. (I'd spent five weeks in the hospital—before and after the birth.) The days and weeks were one long blur. I was breastfeeding on demand, which went fairly well after a few false starts. I learned to always nurse one baby from the right side and the other always on the left. With different demands, I could sometimes be a bit lopsided. But each baby established its own supply. I found it easier to mostly nurse them at the same time.*

"They were nursing almost hourly at first because of their size and then every two hours. Otherwise I would be nursing 24 hours a day! I quickly got the knack of getting them both latched on. Sorting them out when one slips off and starts going crazy with milk spurting everywhere while still trying to hold and nurse the other baby was not so simple.

Sophie screamed loudest. So it just became easier when this happened to take Jules off, restart Sophie and then let Jules resume his feeding. Totally unfair, but it worked."

Tiredness seems to be a constant factor for a mother of twins, especially if there is already a child in the family, as Meg found: *"There were days, especially in the first six weeks, when Joe was at work, going out at 8:30 a.m. and coming home around 10 p.m., when I did not know which way to turn. I remember one evening when both babies were screaming, having nursed all day. Simon was crying on his bed. And I sat on the floor with the babies in my arms and burst into tears myself. It was sheer exhaustion. Most nights I would be up about eight times. They never woke at the same time at night."*

Night feedings may be busier than daytimes. Even when the babies want to sleep, your milk supply may not let you sleep all night.

Pat found she had to keep nursing at night: *"Even when the twins showed all the signs of wanting to stop night feedings, I had to give one of the twins—the hungrier twin—a night feeding. It was too painful for me to go from dusk to dawn without nursing. My milk supply was good. And nursing two babies during the day meant that I would quickly become engorged at night."*

It may come as a surprise to find just how much you need to eat to keep up with your body's needs. Making milk for two (or more) growing babies can consume a vast amount of calories.

Beginning solids, or switching to formula feeding, or both, at around four months, helps some mothers like Pat: *"The twins started to take solids at four months. This was mainly because I found it hard to keep pace with the amount of food I had to eat. I seemed to always be eating. One day I ate a whole family-size chicken for lunch. I followed it with a dessert, then cheese and crackers and hardly felt satisfied. That's when I decided that perhaps I should try solids with the twins."*

Baby rice enabled Hilary to sleep a little longer: *"By nearly four months, we were so tired. My partner and family were begging me to supplement with milk feedings. I was expressing in the morning to give them in the late evening when I was most tired. But the babies were thriving and I really felt bad about 'giving up.' To my relief, my pediatrician suggested a little baby rice in the evening would be better than going to bottles.*

"After rice at about 7 p.m., they would sleep until the late night feeding. Then they went through until 5 or 6 a.m., when we took them into bed and let them help themselves. We swapped babies in between, which was all done half-asleep. This extra sleep was all we needed. I really began to enjoy the whole experience."

The pressure on mothers of twins to wean their babies early can be strong. Many people find it hard to believe that you can provide for all of two babies' needs for any length of time. Olivia resisted the pressure as long as she felt she could: *"At eight months, worries about their weight and comments such as 'Are you sure you have enough milk for them?' finally made me decide to swap to bottles. I do not regret the struggles. I felt that each baby had intimate, almost spiritual, closeness with me. Bottle-feeding would have meant that anyone could have fed them."*

Those who have known the "ups and downs" of breastfeeding twins are, like Hilary, persuasive in their arguments for its benefits: *"I am glad I persevered and still miss it now. Even at the dreadful four-month stage, when we felt there would never be sleep again, I never wished I wasn't breastfeeding. Once they were sleeping a few hours at night, it was truly wonderful."*

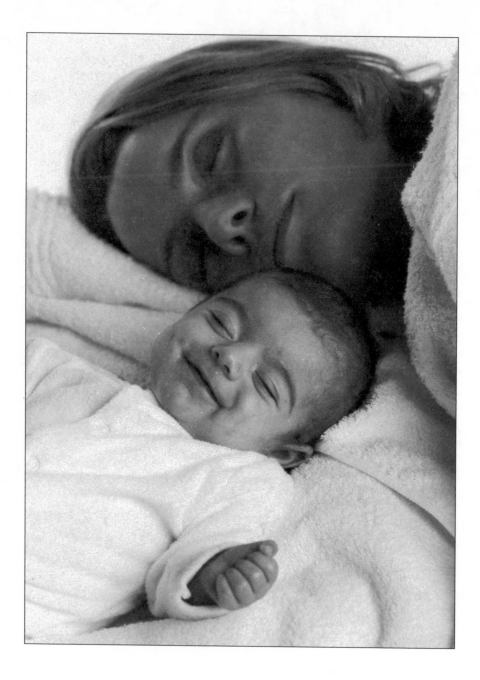

CHAPTER 8   *Breast Troubles*

You may find breastfeeding is truly easy. Problems don't always come up. Some mothers find there are minor troubles to deal with. But for others, major setbacks seem to spell the end of breastfeeding. Almost all problems that arise during breastfeeding have solutions. In many cases, self-help methods are as important as medical interventions. Sometimes self-help is more important to you as you become more aware of how your breasts react. You can often act to prevent problems from getting worse.

As with every other part of child-rearing, lots of people will offer advice. Often it is hard to decide which suggestions are best. The same ideas do not work equally well for every mother, probably because each breastfeeding pair is unique. No one breastfeeds quite like you and your baby do. Your ways may be different than those of other breastfeeding pairs. This does not mean your remedies are better or worse than anyone else's. If they work for you, that's fine. Follow your own instincts and maybe the suggestions offered earlier in this book for dealing with conflicting advice. You will find what works best for you and your baby.

Painful Nipples

There are plenty of horror stories around about women who suffer too much to be able to breastfeed. Some women will hear these sad tales before they begin nursing, as Laura did: *"My own mother breastfed me for six weeks. She had always said that it hurts like being cut with knives the whole time. I had thought that that might happen to me. I knew that I wouldn't put up with that kind of pain."*

FEEDING FILE

Sore and cracked nipples: Some suggestions

- Ask someone you trust to check your baby's position at the breast, especially if your baby is very young.

- Change the position in which you nurse your baby. Try nursing while lying down or with her tucked under your arm.

- Express some milk before putting your baby to the breast. Stimulate your let-down reflex so your baby has less work to do at the start of a feeding.

- Express a little milk after your baby has finished nursing. Gently rub the milk around your nipples and let it dry.

- If you are using creams or ointment, stop using them and see what happens. They may be making the soreness worse.

- Try nursing from the less-sore side first.

- Don't use soap on your nipples. Soap dries the skin.

- Remember to release the suction first if you need to take your baby off the breast.

- If you have been offered a nipple shield, use it as little as possible. Your baby will not be able to take as good a "mouthful"of your breast with the shield. It may increase soreness rather than decrease it. The shield reduces the flow of milk. Long-term use of the shield will reduce your milk supply.

- If your nipples look white or "blanched" when your baby comes off the breast, you may have poor circulation. Some women suffer from Reynaud's syndrome, which may also cause this blanching. Keep your breasts warm and try drinking tea.

In the first seven to 10 days, some women have very sensitive nipples or painful breasts. If the baby is breastfeeding well and nurses whenever he wants, this is usually a short-lived problem. But for some women, like Susy and Leah, the condition lasted for weeks.

"For the first 2½ weeks, I suffered badly from cracked nipples. I never enjoyed nursing. I would put off the dreaded moment until my baby was almost starving! I think the problem perpetuated itself—when my baby was hungry, she sucked even harder. Also, my milk may have flowed less because I felt so tense."

"One suggestion I read was to nurse from the least-sore side first as the baby would suck harder while she was hungry. I found that nursing from the most-sore side first worked better, for me. Ruth liked to play with the nipple near the end of a feeding. Also, with the worst pain over at the beginning, I could relax and enjoy the rest of the feeding."

Without support and good information about positioning, it may be hard to find a nursing position that is not painful to your breasts. Women try all sorts of things to find some relief for their pain. Elaine experimented: *"I tried most things—hot washcloths, going topless, expressing with a pump (agony), lanolin, and rubbing my breast milk on my nipples. I also tried different positions and taking my baby off of my breast until the latch looked OK. But both my husband and I found it hard to see his lower lip. The more things I tried, the more frustrated and angry he got."*

Fortunately, skilled, sensitive support is there if you need it, as Hilary discovered: *"The nipples both cracked. When I got home after five days, nursing became even more painful. I got shaky before a feeding because I knew it was going to hurt so much. David would get upset. I would get upset. Matthew was such a great help to me at this time. He calmed us both down and got me to contact a lactation consultant. I was surprised that she was prepared to see us right away. She watched how I nursed David. Then she helped me get more comfortable and David in a better position. We tried several times before there was any difference. But I felt so much more relaxed! Here was someone who seemed to know what she was doing. She made me feel as if she would sit there all night with me if necessary. It was so reassuring.*

"Finally we found a position where David began to nurse and it just didn't hurt. I really didn't believe it was possible until it happened. It was wonderful. A lot more talk with the consultant, reassurance, and such, and we went home. It was harder at home. But since I knew it was possible for it not to hurt, I was prepared to take David off and try again until it worked. It took about a week for the cracks to heal on both sides."

Sometimes nipple shields are offered to mothers with sore nipples. The shields may help the pain and enable the crack to heal. But they don't change the source of the problem. They may also create new problems. The breast cannot be milked as well through a shield. Your baby will not be able to take as large a mouthful of breast as he can without it; thus, the baby receives less milk at each feeding. Over time, the mother's milk supply may be reduced.[51,52] After a while, some babies refuse to nurse without the shield when it is removed.

Janice found nipple shields a mixed blessing: *"I couldn't see why my nipples had cracked. Michael's latch looked right but felt wrong. Perhaps his small mouth didn't open wide enough. Maybe I was hold-*

ing him along the wrong arm. The nurse suggested I use nipple shields until the nipples healed. It took four days. I was eager to resume direct breastfeeding. I was concerned that Michael might forget how to latch on to the breast. I started back on the breast a little at a time. Four days later, just as I stopped using the shields, my nipples cracked again. I solved the problem when I completely changed the way I held Michael."

To Liza, shields seemed to be the perfect answer, until she found some of the hidden drawbacks: *"When my first baby was born, the nurse fixed me up with a nipple shield to help my baby breastfeed the first few days. No one warned me that my baby would become so used to the shield that he would reject the nipple. On top of this, the nipple shield seemed to cut down the amount of milk my baby was getting."*

Bethan found she needed the nipple shields. It took her a long time to manage without them: *"The nipple shield is amazing, in more ways than one. Yes, I can now nurse on the sore side with the shield. But I can also see now that the nipple is actually bleeding during a feeding. I find the sight of bloody milk collecting in the shield while the baby comes up for air very disturbing. Nursing at home continues with relative comfort using the shield. My nurse tried to convince me that 48 hours is long enough for the crack to heal, and that the baby wouldn't nurse well enough with the shield. So I tried nursing without it. The pain reduced me to such a state of distress that the nurse almost fled in embarrassment. In fact, it took almost two weeks before I could think about trying without the shield and three weeks to say that I was OK again. I am now just over seven weeks into motherhood and still breastfeeding. I nurse about eight times a day—and usually use the shield on either side at least once a day."*

Thrush

Nipple soreness may develop due to reasons other than positioning, such as thrush or dermatitis (inflamed skin). You might need help from a health provider or a lactation consultant to learn the cause of the problem and to find an effective solution.

Pam's son Scott developed oral thrush: *"Antibiotics were prescribed at the hospital for an infection of his navel. The thrush didn't bother him at all. But it did need to be treated. This meant giving Scott drops four*

BACKGROUND NOTES

Thrush

Many people have the kind of yeast on their skin that causes thrush infection *candida albicans.* Most of the time the yeast is inactive and not noticeable, but sometimes it multiplies and causes infections. Antibiotics kill bacteria, but they may also kill the bacteria that help prevent yeast infections. They do not kill the yeast, so it multiplies freely. Thrush infections develop more often if you are under stress, eat a poor diet, or are run-down or anemic. Thrush is passed easily from mother to baby, or from baby to mother.

Signs of thrush

- On the nipple—white spots on the nipple, red and sore nipples that do not clear up, and itching, scaly skin.
- In the baby's mouth—white spots that do not rub off.
- A sore red diaper rash may be a sign of thrush.
- Pain deep in the breast, throbbing in the breast between feedings, and pain while nursing may be signs of thrush in the milk ducts.

What may help

- Thrush likes alkaline conditions, so don't use soap. Use neutral cleansers or plain water.
- A teaspoon of baking soda in a cup of warm water makes a weak acid wash. Use this on your nipples. It may help get rid of thrush.
- A tablespoon of vinegar in a glass of water can also have this effect.
- Natural, live yogurt contains bacteria that act against thrush. Smooth it on your nipples. It can be soothing.
- Keep the nipples dry. Thrush likes moist, warm places.

When to seek medical help

- As soon you suspect thrush. Thrush is not likely to clear up without medical treatment.

What a doctor might do

- Prescribe antifungal cream, gel or drops.
- Treat both mother and baby, even if only one has symptoms. If just one of the pair is treated, chances are good that the thrush will come back.
- Recommend applying antifungal medications to the nipple for thrush in the milk duct. Some people have found that a course of antifungal Nystatin pills works for thrush in the ducts.
- Precribe a course of treatment that lasts several weeks. Thrush is persistent. A longer course of treatment helps make sure it won't come back right away.

Keep it from coming back

- If thrush comes back, check other places where thrush may be found, such as the vagina or the baby's bottom. The whole family may need treatment.
- Don't use antibiotics if possible. If you must use them, take antifungal treatment at the same time.

times a day and putting cream on my nipples twice a day. The thrush came back a few times. Finally, after several courses of treatment, a hospital visit and a hefty dose of treatment for both of us, we got rid of it. I am susceptible to getting thrush, but seven months into nursing my second baby it has not occurred at all."

Once thrush has been identified, both you and your baby must be treated. Thrush likes warm, moist places. A mother's nipple in a baby's mouth provides the perfect medium for growth. Sometimes the treatment may take some time, as it did for Jane with her third baby: *"At six weeks, my nipples became a bit sore. I looked in the baby's mouth and saw white spots. Two prescriptions of Nystatin® drops failed to get it. Then I got gentian violet for the baby's mouth, which worked almost overnight. I used Lansinoh® cream on my nipples. A doctor friend suggested this, not my pediatrician."*

Jane also got thrush when her fourth baby was very young: *"My nipples got worse instead of better. By day 10 I was in tears at every feeding, the pain was so bad. I thought about thrush. But I was so tired I dismissed it. I thought we couldn't have got it this early—from where? A friend asked me if I had looked in the baby's mouth. I hadn't.*

"The next day we had our visit with the pediatrician. We looked and found lots of white spots. The baby had been difficult to latch on—no wonder! I looked at my nipples later. I couldn't believe I hadn't noticed the mess they were in. Bright pink fiery skin all over the nipples and radiating out over the areola—like star shapes.

"My pediatrician prescribed oral gel for Claire's mouth—nothing for me! I used the cream I had from a previous bout of thrush after feedings. I also used vinegar solution sometimes and gave my nipples a lot of fresh air. I used nipple shields, but they barely took the edge off the pain. The thrush cleared up after about a week. It was great to enjoy nursing finally! It did come back a few weeks later. But I noticed it quickly and still had the cream and gel ready to use."

Other Causes of Soreness

Sometimes soreness is caused by other skin conditions, such as dermatitis or eczema. These can be harder to treat, as Jennifer learned: *"We got off to a bad start with sore nipples, which became sore areola. After treating us for thrush, they learned I had eczema. I had to use hydrocortisone cream which, of course, had to be washed off before each*

*Use gravity to help
the milk flow.*

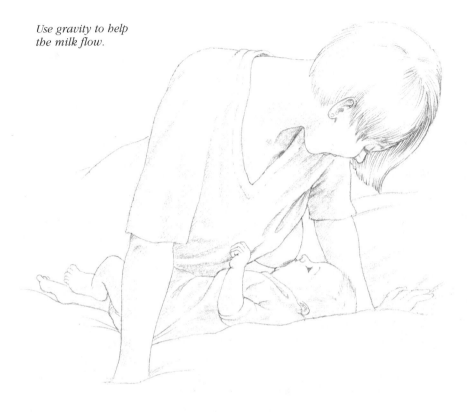

*feeding. By the time my baby was seven months old, my skin was better.
I gradually managed to do without the hydrocortisone."*

Sometimes you may find your nipples become sore again, once the
early days of nursing are over. There could be several reasons. Your
baby may be teething. Her saliva may be more acid for a while. You
may be pregnant. You may be about to resume menstruation. Whatever
the cause, it almost never lasts very long.

Jennifer describes her symptoms and the surprise she got when she
learned the cause: *"When Carol was about nine months old, I started to
find nursing her really painful again. It was very much as it was in the
early days. It hurt enough for me to be swearing or nearly in tears when
she wanted to nurse. I wondered whether I might be pregnant. I actually tried a home pregnancy test. A few days later, I had the start of my
first period since she had been conceived."*

Painful Breasts

Blocked Ducts and Mastitis

Sometimes one or more of the milk ducts becomes blocked. This may happen all at once, after weeks of trouble-free breastfeeding. You can feel a lump, which may be tender. These lumps are caused by a blocked duct. The blockage prevents the milk from flowing. Common causes of blocked ducts are too-tight bras, sleeping in a bra or sleeping with your arm in an awkward position across your breast. Or you might have gotten bruised from cuddling a bouncy toddler. Blocked ducts need prompt treatment, or they can lead to *mastitis* (a swollen breast). Happily, they respond well to self-help.

Sheila found nursing her baby was the best cure: *"Just when I was getting the hang of things, I started to get blocked ducts. This was painful for me—definitely the worst thing about breastfeeding. I had lumps, very tender and sometimes covering a third of the breast for two to three days. I used a warm compress and painful massaging. I tried a breast pump with little success. Often the lump would go away while Helen was nursing.*

"Sometimes I would have a lump a week. I got depressed. This continued for four months. I was very close to giving up. Just when some people seemed to stop nursing (about four months) things started to go well. I began to enjoy it."

Sometimes self-help works well, as it did for Jean: *"I still had to be careful of blocked ducts if I used breast shields too often, or wore a smaller bra. But the second time this happened, I kept it from getting worse by using arm-swinging exercises, and 'combing' my soaped breast. These were ideas the lactation consultant had given me."*

You may find that you develop a blockage at the very end of your nipple. It can look like a pimple or a blister. This can be from milk solids that have built up in a blocked duct. They can be stubborn to remove. You may need special treatment to remove them as well as the usual self-help techniques.

Carol used her knowledge as a lactation consultant: *"I noticed a slightly tender place in my right breast. It was just behind the areola. I found a tiny white blister, no bigger than a pinhead, on the nipple. I could pierce the blister with a sterile needle, but I was in a lot of pain by then and didn't want to try it. I didn't want the pain to get worse. It could*

BACKGROUND NOTES

Blocked Ducts

Signs of a blockage

- A lump you can see or feel
- A tender area
- Milk solids coming from the nipple as a small white spot. Or, a white blister on the nipple.

What may help

- Nurse the baby first from the "lumpy" side.
- Nurse with the baby's chin nearest to the lump. This way his lower jaw can strip the lump better.
- Use gravity to help the milk flow. Lay the baby on his back and hang the lumpy breast over him.
- Massage the breast gently.
- Warmth may help the milk flow.
- Use a wide-tooth comb covered with soap or baby oil and firm but gentle pressure to stroke the breast over the lump towards the nipple.
- Express milk after a feeding if the breast still feels lumpy.

- A white spot or blister on the nipple may need extra attention from your healthcare provider.

Has it worked?

- The lump should begin to get smaller and less tender.
- It may take a few days to disappear.

When to seek medical help

- Within a few days, if the lump does not respond to any of the treatment options above.

Keep it from coming back

- Check bra and clothing. Make sure they are not too tight and do not put pressure on the breast tissue.
- Check baby's position at the breast.
- Check that your fingers don't press into breast tissue when nursing.
- Change nursing positions regularly.
- Don't wear a bra in bed.

---

have been caused by a blocked duct. Nearby, my breast was becoming lumpy, though neither hot nor red, thank goodness. So I did what I would normally do for a blocked duct and hoped it would get better soon! Sure enough, within three or four days it was better. The blister had burst and dried up in the process."

If you don't treat blocked ducts, your breasts may swell or you may get mastitis. Mastitis can strike suddenly. It may also start slowly, often from a simple blockage. Mastitis simply means *inflammation of the breast*. It does not mean there is an infection in the breast, but there may be. If you go to your doctor with symptoms of mastitis, you may be given an antibiotic, because infection can spread quickly. Your doctor will want to prevent an abscess (infection) from forming.

BACKGROUND NOTES

Mastitis

Mastitis is inflammation. It is not always infection. Milk from a blocked duct may have leaked into the breast tissue. The body may think this is an infection and react in the same way by increasing the blood supply to the area, which produces swelling and redness. Infection in the breast looks the same as inflammation. You cannot tell if there is an infection unless you check the milk for the presence of bacteria.

Signs of mastitis

- Red inflamed place on the breast (or whole breast)
- Breast feels sore
- You have flu-like symptoms—aches, shivers, fever, feel tired and emotional

What may help

- Keep on breastfeeding. Don't stop even if you are told to. Not nursing can make mastitis worse.
- Nurse the baby more often. Use a breast pump if the baby is not taking all the milk.
- Nurse first from the sore side.
- Use the advice for treating a blocked duct.
- Exercise to help stimulate the circulation. Swing your arms. (Scrubbing the floor or washing windows can help as well.)
- Rest if you feel ill.
- Alternate warmth and cold. Use warm washcloths or warm water splashed on breasts, or a warm shower or bath, especially before a feeding. Try cold compresses (a package of frozen peas or ice-cubes wrapped in a clean dishtowel are good) after a feeding to help the swelling go down.

Has it worked?

- Self-help techniques should work in 12 to 24 hours.
- Flu-like feelings and swelling should ease.

When to seek medical help

- If self-help techniques don't help in 12 to 24 hours (or sooner if you are worried).
- If mastitis keeps coming back.

What a doctor might do

- Prescribe antibiotics. Make sure it's one you can take while breastfeeding. You do not have to stop breastfeeding while taking most antibiotics.
- Baby may get cranky or develop diarrhea from antibiotics in the milk. It isn't harmful, but the baby may want more frequent feedings if she is thirsty.
- Some mothers find that eating live yogurt helps prevent thrush that can sometimes result from taking antibiotics.

How to keep it from coming back

- Check the position of the baby at the breast.
- Change feeding positions regularly.
- Cut down on saturated fats (those that are solid at room temperature, such as butter, lard, some peanut butters). Stay away from caffeine (including tea, coffee, cola drinks, chocolate).
- Don't use sprays or creams on your nipples. They may affect the skin's natural barriers.
- If mastitis comes back more than twice, ask your doctor to take a swab from the baby's nose and throat. The baby may have an infection, which reinfects you.

Combing the breast to help clear a blocked duct.

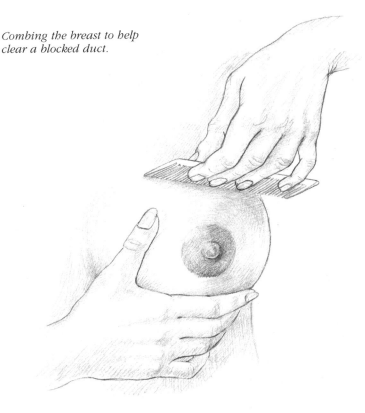

The best way to treat mastitis is to increase the amount of milk flowing through the breast. You can do this by nursing the baby more often. If you stop breastfeeding at this time you will only make matters worse.[34] You can treat mastitis with the same self-help remedies that work for a blocked duct. But you may need to take antibiotics as well. Sometimes, though, taking antibiotics can lead to more problems for your baby as well as for you.

If you have mastitis, you'll feel terrible for awhile. Julia remembers: *"When Susan was five months old, I got mastitis. I felt fine all day. We had friends over in the evening. But when they got up to leave, I couldn't move! I tried all the self-help remedies I could and kept nursing. I went to see the doctor the next morning. He was very understanding. He said to keep on with the self-help but also prescribed antibiotics. He told me not to use them unless I really needed them, because they would be passed through to the milk.*

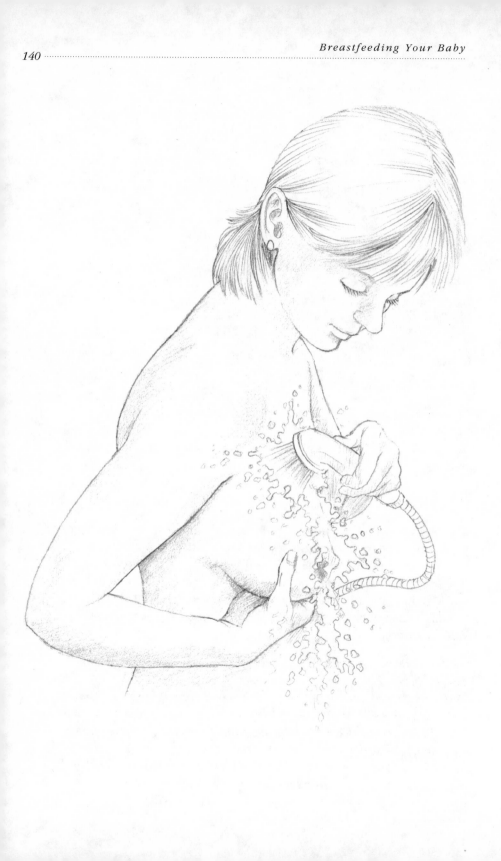

"By that evening, I felt so bad that I started taking the antibiotics. Within 24 hours, Susan was miserable, had diarrhea and a bad diaper rash. The mastitis soon cleared up. But Susan's diaper rash got so bad that it bled at diaper changes.

"I took her to the doctor's. She had gotten thrush. The doctor prescribed cream to apply at diaper changes. Over the next four months, the thrush continued. We had to make three more trips to the doctor for different creams. Had I realized the extent of the damage that the antibiotics could cause, I would have tried to avoid them."

If you get mastitis, you may only get it once while you are breastfeeding. Some mothers get it several times. If you do, try to learn the cause. Sometimes an infection in the baby's nose can infect you if it is not noticed.

Some mothers become good at spotting the first signs of mastitis. They manage to clear it up without needing to take antibiotics, like Jackie: *"While nursing Molly, I had mastitis twice, at nine and 13 weeks. I think it was because of a small bra and a sudden increase in my milk supply. After the second attack of mastitis, I talked to a counselor. She had me try changing nursing positions to help drain all parts of the breast and to express milk if I was very full. A hand pump was useless. But I learned to express by hand, leaning over a sterilized ice-cube tray. The let down did all the work! By then, I was always looking for lumps. This led to some very strange nursing positions (not possible in public!). If I felt full, I would often not wear my bra. I kept nursing Molly happily until she was nine months old, when she weaned herself."*

Sore Breasts

Sometimes may feel that your whole breast is sore and painful, but you don't seem to have the symptoms of mastitis. These pains may be due to thrush in the milk ducts, which can cause pain deep in the breast. Sometimes there doesn't seem to be an obvious cause. You may really have mastitis, diagnosed only after you have struggled on in pain for some time. This is more likely if you have suffered sore nipples.

It is easy to think the mastitis is just more nipple and breast soreness, as Amy did: *"My nipples cracked on both breasts. Nursing was torture. Deep pains seemed to start in my armpits and spread through my whole breast. This lasted the whole feeding. I often cried while nursing, it was so painful—or before, just thinking of the pain. I tried most things—hot washcloths, going topless, expressing with a pump. I also tried different positions and taking my baby off my breast until the latch looked OK. The turning point came when I went home to my parents for Christmas. My baby was about three weeks old. My mother insisted I see a doctor because my breast was inflamed. I was diagnosed as having mastitis and antibiotics were prescribed. Within a few days, the deep pain within my breasts eased and latching on became much easier. By six weeks, I still had pain but just on latching. By eight weeks, I was nursing pain-free. Two years and three months later, I am still nursing Timothy."*

Abscess

A breast abcess is no fun. Any mother who finds she has one may need a few weeks to recover. Sometimes, an abscess responds to antibiotics without further treatment. But more often, the abscess is lanced and drained in the hospital. Sometimes it may be *aspirated* (the pus is drawn out). Jayne's experience is typical: *"After about seven weeks, I got a breast abscess. Before I knew that's what it was, I struggled through more and more pain. I thought I had a blocked duct. Finally I was driven to the doctor, who diagnosed mastitis. After three courses of antibiotics and a lot of pain, I was in the hospital. The abscess was so large it needed to be drained surgically. Then there were two weeks of daily visits to the hospital. After that, [I had to go] three times a week to the clinic before I was down to a simple bandage. The whole time I wanted to take a shower without having to worry about getting the bandage wet."*

Blood in the Milk or Colostrum

Rarely during pregnancy, you may notice streaks of blood in the colostrum that leaks from your breasts. If there is a lot of blood, the colostrum may look like cold tea or coffee. For some women, this may continue after the birth without any nipple soreness or cracks.

Nadine was 16 weeks pregnant when her breasts started to leak: *"Shortly after this, I was horrified to find what looked like blood in the colostrum. I was especially concerned because only one breast was affected to begin with. I imagined all sorts of dreadful things. When the second breast also started to 'bleed,' I felt relieved. It seemed more likely to have to do with pregnancy than cancer, if they were both doing it."*

BACKGROUND NOTES

Abscess

An abscess may come from poorly treated blocked ducts or mastitis, especially if you have stopped breastfeeding. You can get an abscess without any other symptoms.

Signs of an abscess

- A soft lump may be felt on breast
- The lump may or may not be painful
- Pus may be seen in the milk
- Not feeling well, as with mastitis

What may help

- Keep breastfeeding, as long as the baby is not sick from blood or pus in the milk.
- Express milk from affected side. Keep nursing from other side to maintain supply.

When to seek medical help

- Right away! An abscess is a medical condition that needs quick treatment.

What a doctor might do

- Prescribe antibiotics
- Lance and drain the abscess
- Aspirate the abscess (insert a syringe and draw off the fluids inside). This may be done once or twice. Aspiration is an alternative to lancing and draining.
- Aspiration is less traumatic and may disrupt breastfeeding less.

How to keep it from coming back

- If the abscess results from blocked ducts or mastitis, follow suggestions above for these conditions.
- Don't wean quickly. Wean slowly, over a few weeks.

Blood in the milk or colostrum can be alarming. There is not much written about it in the breastfeeding literature. Some doctors may not know what to make of it. You might think think the worst, as Lilian did: *"Two days after the birth of my first child I noticed, to my horror, blood in the colostrum from my left breast. I told the nurse right away. No one seemed to have seen this problem before. The staff had nothing helpful to say. In fact, their negative response made me even more scared. I was convinced something was very wrong with me."*

Sandy also received little help or reassurance: *"I was upset. I felt worse after talking to one of the nurses. She said that blood in the milk would make breastfeeding impossible because the baby would be sick all the time. During labor, one or two nurses were startled to see 'blood' on my hospital gown long before my son was born. One went away and looked*

in her textbooks. She came back to tell me that it was called a red-colored discharge and not blood. Another said she had seen it only once before in her career."

Most women find the blood goes away as soon as the milk comes in. They begin to breastfeed normally. Your baby will not be harmed by the blood. However, if you or your partner have had multiple sexual partners or have used IV drugs, do get checked for HIV. Mothers with HIV are advised not to breastfeed to prevent transmitting the disease to the baby.

Some women, like Liz, are told to express and then throw out milk from the affected breast: *"The nurse was helpful. She got me to use the electric breast pump on the affected side until the milk was clear of the blood. But she told me to keep on nursing from the right breast. Once my milk came in, the blood began to disappear. A final sample of my milk showed that I could now nurse from both sides. What a relief!"*

Allie reassured the nurses, rather than the other way around: *"After my son was born he was put to my breast right away. We quickly succeeded in breastfeeding. He didn't have any problems with the taste as far as I could tell. And he was not a 'sickly' baby at all. I had to reassure the nurses a few times, because once in a while, when he did bring milk back up after a feeding in the first few days, it was an orangey-brown color! Luckily, when the milk came in, it was normal and the 'bleeding' stopped."*

Blood in your milk or colostrum may be similar to a nosebleed. The cells lining the milk ducts are fed by fragile *capillaries* (tiny blood vessels). Some of these may burst on their own. Or they may be broken from expressing colostrum too vigorously. Rarely, the blood does not "clear up." In this case, check with a doctor to see if there is any cause for concern.

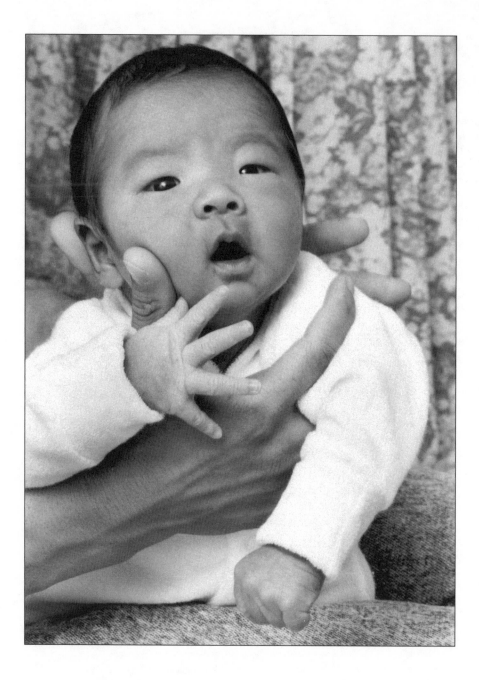

CHAPTER 9 *Nursing Problems*

Sometimes breastfeeding itself seems to be going well, but your baby becomes cranky or fussy. You may wonder if you are doing something wrong. You may worry that your breast milk is not "enough" for your baby. These are common concerns when you provide all your baby's nutrition. In many cases, there is no real answer. Babies are people and have moods and feelings like anybody else. They are very good at expressing themselves, loudly! Sometimes you will make a connection from their crying to breastfeeding. Once you spot the problem, you can often handle it. Be patient and keep trying.

Crying Babies

In the early weeks at home, you begin to understand and interpret your baby's "language." You try to learn how to respond to the cries of your baby. When you respond to the baby's cries, you expect the crying to stop—that's natural. It is distressing to hear a baby cry. Perhaps we think that, as parents, we will can always find the magic cure.

It seems as though there is some pressure on new parents to find the "cure" for crying quickly. Relatives might ask, "Has the baby settled down yet?" This could be another way of asking, have you figured out your baby? Can you respond to the baby so that there is not too much crying? People really seem to want "things to settle down" after the birth of a baby.

In most cases, "things" do get easier after the first couple of weeks. But for some parents, they do not. If you have to listen to the sound of your baby crying, knowing a list of possible fixes does not console the baby or you. It can be a hard time. Luckily for most parents, times of persistent crying are few. For others, they do go on longer and cause a lot of stress for everyone concerned.

Mary had a rough time: *"Everything was fine until she was about three weeks old. Then she began to scream all night long, nursing on and off. She would only stop crying when she was rocked. She would nurse and settle down for a short while and then begin screaming again. This was a hard time for me. I wish I had known about lactation counselors and La Leche League. However, I kept going. I knew that I was doing the right thing by breastfeeding although I was often advised to stop. My mother-in-law told me I should put her on the bottle because my milk was obviously too thin.*

"I took Liz to the clinic regularly and was assured by my pediatrician that she was fine. Her weight gain was certainly enough, sometimes 1 pound in a week. I badly needed reassurance that there was nothing wrong with my milk supply or the baby. Luckily help was there. As time went on, Liz still screamed most of the night. The nurse advised me to limit nursing to three-hour intervals to keep her from stimulating my milk supply too much and giving herself a tummy ache. I tried to get help from my pediatrician. But again I only got reassurance that my baby was healthy. He didn't offer any other advice or solutions. I resented the attitude that my problems were the result of my incompetence. I still felt that I was doing the right thing.

"Finally, things did improve. She screamed less, nursed less and slept more. The improvement came slowly. I tried to solve my own problems by reading as much as I could about nursing and crying babies. I was never able to figure out the cause of Liz's crying. I wonder if she was allergic to dairy products she got through my milk. It was hard to cut these foods out of my diet. I didn't work at that for very long. I still don't know whether Liz had colic or a stomach ache or if I just had too much milk."

Mary searched for an answer she didn't find. Luckily, she was able to keep breastfeeding. She held on to the belief that breastfeeding was the right thing for her and her baby. Not all women can be so confident about breastfeeding when faced with an unhappy baby. This seems to be very closely bound up with their own confidence and self-esteem.

FEEDING FILE

How to comfort a crying baby

- Offer the breast, for comfort if not for food.

- Tiny babies need to suck. Some babies need more sucking time than others. You may wish to try a pacifier. But you should know that sometimes pacifiers can affect a small baby's ability to suck at the breast.

- Give her a clean finger to suck for a while.

- Hold your baby near you. Your heart-beat is a comforting sound. Some babies like to be held upright, near your shoulder.

- Many babies like movement. Try a rocking chair, or simple, natural rocking that men and women do when holding a baby.

- Your baby may like the gentle rhythm of patting or stroking. Caress your baby to help him feel secure.

- Some babies like to be swaddled, an age-old practice. Lay the baby on a shawl, soft blanket or sheet. Wrap him snugly, with each arm held down next to his body.

- Warm water may help him relax. Give him a bath alone. Or, even better, nurse him while you have a warm bath together.

- Show him his reflection in a mirror. Babies love to look at faces. The mirror will give him a new view of his mother or father.

- The gentle sound of his parents' voices can be soothing.

- Offer a different view or experience to your baby. Try a ride in the car or watching the washing machine spin, for example.

- A noise, like a vacuum cleaner, can soothe some cranky babies. Others may respond to womb-music tapes if you try them in the early weeks.

- An older baby may enjoy kicking on a mat without his diaper.

- An older baby may like to sit in a bouncy cradle-type chair and watch his parents.

- She may like to lie in a stroller in the garden. The leaves and clouds may be soothing to watch. Be sure to protect her from too much sun.

- Sometimes your baby may cry because she wants to sleep, but is just too tired to be able to "let go." Hold her close, speak or sing gently and stay calm. This may help her get to sleep.

- If you become upset by her crying, place her safely in crib or a stroller. Leave her for a few minutes while you calm down.

- Ask for some help, so you can have "time off."

- Phone a friend or a breastfeeding counselor and talk about how you feel.

- If it all seems to be getting out of control, contact a self-help support group. The following contacts may be able to provide a referral: your health provider, La Leche League leader, county Health Department (in the United States), provincial or territorial Health Ministry (in Canada), church or temple.

- Ask your doctor for advice.

- If you think your baby may be sensitive to dairy products in your diet, ask a breastfeeding counselor about how to eat well while cutting out dairy products.

The view of motherhood that many women have is often composed of fairly vague memories of their own mothers, mixed with very powerful images from the media. Media images are pretty clear. A happy, contented baby means a "good" mother. A woman coping with a crying baby very easily seems the opposite. An unhappy, crying baby means a "bad" mother. This can be demoralizing. You may believe that somehow the baby's crying is really *your* fault. A comment, for example, that the baby is crying because of the "nature" of your milk could make you think about giving up breastfeeding completely. Even if you know that it is not the case, it can feel like too much "blame" to carry.

Colic

Some people may suggest that your baby's crying is caused by "colic" or a stomach ache. No one really knows what might cause the type of crying that is often described as "screaming." This crying does seem to be of a different quality. It sounds to parents as though their baby is in pain.

Sometimes, an answer can relieve you, even though you still have to cope with a crying baby, as Nina did: *"My son Josh, now nearly six months old, suffered from 'colic' for the first 12 weeks of his life. At first I enjoyed the closeness I felt when nursing Josh. But as his colic got worse, I felt guilty, as if it was my fault that he was in so much pain. I wondered if there was something wrong with my milk. I went to the doctor with him lots of times, because I was concerned that there might be something else wrong with him. He cried day and night (well, not quite, but it felt like it!).*

"The doctor explained that she thought that, because he was a big baby (he was 9 lb. 1 oz. at birth), he would get very hungry and gulp his milk but also take in a lot of air. (I have to add that he never burped, no matter how much we tried to burp him.) This was also part of the problem. He would start to nurse and after just a few minutes he would start to cry. That showed me he couldn't take much milk. I began to feel desperate.

"Plenty of people told me to 'put him on the bottle' and that he was just hungry. But I didn't believe this was the case (I still don't). I did get very upset sometimes when nursing him, he was so unhappy and fussy. My husband and I used to take turns walking around the room carrying him. It didn't seem to help Josh much. At least we felt we were doing

something to try to comfort him. Anyway, I am glad to say that all seems a long time ago—he is a happy little guy now. When we were told that this was sometimes called three-month colic . . . *well, the three months seemed to take a lot longer than that!"*

Does persistent crying occur mostly in the evening? This may be the busiest time of day for you. Some researchers suggest that the baby may cry at this time because he is not getting all that he needs in the way of food or comfort from you while you are busy with household chores. You might be extra busy if you have older children to care for. Some women figure this out by themselves and adjust their way of life accordingly.

Paula did just that: *"Some evenings I found Charlotte very fussy, crying, eager to nurse but refusing the breast. This, of course, is typical behavior in young babies. After some weeks I found an answer: I figured out that if I had skimped on my lunch or missed a snack in the afternoon, then Charlotte would yell the house down at night.*

"I expect most of us find late afternoon and early evening a busy time. Sometimes it can even be a frantic time of day. I know I can feel wiped out by dinnertime! To overcome this low, I always ate a good-sized snack when I came home with Hannah from school. I fixed my evening meal earlier in the day. Or else I bought easy, ready-made meals. I did any urgent tasks earlier in the day if I could. Or else I just left them. This helped me slow the pace at the end of the day."

You may seek want to seek the advice of your healthcare providers. You may be concerned that there might be something wrong with the baby.

Colette was able to link events after reading about possible food allergies: *"At about 10 days, Luke got severe infant colic. Like most first-time parents, we had never heard of this. We were terrified to find that it seemed there was nothing we could do about it. We tried medicines to help the baby's digestion. None seemed to help.*

"My doctor could only suggest that I shouldn't eat spicy foods. My breastfeeding counselor offered her sympathies. My mother told me about someone who had had a similar problem, and found that it was caused by dairy products in her own diet. I gave up milk, cheese and many other things. Within a week, the colic was gone. Every time I drank even a tiny bit of milk, the colic came back. It would start about 24 hours after I had eaten the offending substance and take about three

days to go. During that time, Luke would scream in agony each evening. Sometimes he wouldn't stop till 5 a.m. the next morning. In the end, I gave up all dairy products until Luke was weaned at eight months. I did not find this too hard. In fact, cow's milk now tastes very strange! But I did miss cheese—our diet is mostly vegetarian. This adjustment was a small price to pay for a colic-free baby, I thought.

"My main problem with the dairy-free diet was other people's attitudes. My doctor just would not believe that milk was to blame for the colic. She kept on suggesting other possible causes—spices, orange juice, grapes. I learned that some health providers and childbirth educators had known about the link between dairy products and colic for some time, but they had not mentioned it to me as a possible cause. A Canadian friend recently passed on an article from a healthcare journal citing research that indicates at least one-third of babies with colic will show significant improvement if their mothers give up milk.[51] I feel that if people who knew about this had told me from the beginning, I could have saved Luke many weeks of pain, and my husband and I would've had fewer sleepless nights.

"My breastfeeding counselor did give me a helpful diet sheet—after I learned the cause of the colic. It explained the importance of maintaining a good intake of calcium on a dairy-free diet. For eight months, I ate tons of sesame seeds and sardines—but not together! I wanted to make sure Luke's bones grew well. And I didn't want to get osteoporosis."

Babies born to families with a history of allergies are more likely to be sensitive to various substances. Cow's milk is one of the most likely allergens. Exposure to the allergen can cause some sort of reaction—often a fussy, unhappy baby. It could be that your baby received a bottle of cow's milk formula in the hospital, or as an early supplement. This can be enough to sensitize the baby to the cow's milk substances in your breast milk, if you eat dairy products. If this is the case, cut out all dairy products from your diet. This may bring a great deal of relief to you and your baby. If you think your baby may be reacting to something in your diet, it might help to talk to your pediatrician or a dietitian.

It may be that a crying baby is sensitive to something he is taking into his stomach. This could be directly, such as vitamin drops. Or it could be something that passed through your milk, such as the vitamins or iron tablets you are taking. Faced with a crying baby, many women keep close track of what the baby receives. Caffeine is often cited as a possible stimulant. If you drink more than five cups of drinks that contain caffeine each day, you baby might become more "fussy" than usual. (Coffee, tea, many soft drinks and chocolate contain caffeine.) After it is cut out of your diet, it takes about two weeks to be sure a substance is gone from your breast milk. Stick with it and exclude the substance from your diet to see if it irritates your baby. It is sensible to discuss any exclusion diet with your doctor, pediatrician, or dietitian before starting. They may have useful advice for you. Lactation counselors may also provide you with helpful information.

If your baby's stools are always watery and green and she is not gaining weight well even though you seem to have plenty of milk, she might be getting too much foremilk and not enough hindmilk. The watery foremilk is rich in lactose. Too much lactose makes breastmilk pass through the baby too quickly.[54] She needs to receive both the foremilk and the fatty high-calorie hindmilk. Try to let her finish the first breast before offering the second. Later on, she may prefer to take just one breast at each feeding.

There may not be an easy "answer" to your baby's crying. Some babies seem to cry despite every effort to calm them. The more support and encouragement you receive the better. This difficult phase of your baby's life will pass.

Breast Refusal

One of the most distressing experiences a breastfeeding mother can have is when her baby suddenly refuses to nurse from the breast. Sometimes this happens after months of happy nursing. It can seem as if the baby is rejecting her mother, not just the breastfeeding, as Annabel recalls: *"My milk seemed to let down with great force, especially on one side. Tracey would pull away choking and gasping for breath. Then she would often refuse to nurse again for some time, she was so upset. This made me feel like a real failure. I wanted nursing to be a happy time for both of us. Instead I felt as if I were torturing my baby."*

When Lee's baby, Simon, was nine months old, he had six teeth. He was so proud of them that he started trying them out while nursing. One day he bit really hard and Lee reacted by saying "No!": *"The next day, Simon nursed as usual. But the day after that he would not nurse at all. He would burst into tears when I tried to latch him on. He became very upset. At first I wasn't sure what the cause might be. I thought through everything—a change in the taste of the milk, the smell. Finally I decided it must have been my reaction when Simon bit me.*

"Over the next few days we both became very upset. I worried that I might have put him off nursing completely. I expressed milk to give him from a cup, because I wanted to maintain my supply. I had several comments from people trying to be helpful, such as: 'He's nine months old. Perhaps it's a good time to wean him.' I know they meant well, but these comments did not help. I wasn't ready to wean him yet. Why do people always assume that mothers are looking for an excuse to stop breastfeeding once the baby is six months old? I persevered and gave Simon a lot of love and cuddling. Finally, on day five, he began to nurse again as if nothing had happened. Simon is now nearing his first birthday and is still nursing three times a day."

Your baby may refuse to nurse after an upset, such as Lee describes. Or he may simply refuse to nurse. He may kick and scream, and fight you as you try to offer him your breast. Each feeding can become harder. This may last for a few days. Sudden refusal of the breast like this is not often a sign that your baby is ready to be weaned from the breast. He may be upset, but it can be hard to spot the reason.

Sometimes, your baby may be ill. Lee describes how her son reacted: *"When my second child was eight months old, he became ill. He refused all food and fluids, including breast milk. He became dehydrated and was in the hospital. Most of the health providers I saw at that time did not understand why I was so upset at his refusal of the breast. But I felt that the most natural way to comfort my child was to breastfeed him. It was agony to see him screaming in pain and not be able to comfort him. Finally the problem was diagnosed as a bad strep infection in the throat. It was so bad that he couldn't swallow. By this time he had not nursed for five days. Although he received treatment that helped him very quickly, he now connected the breast with pain. He screamed if I lifted my blouse to nurse him. This was really upsetting. I wanted very much to try to get him back on to the breast.*

"At first I just held him next to my breast when he was asleep. Then, over a few days, I would put the nipple near his mouth and express a few drops on to his lips as he slept. Finally, one day he latched on in his sleep. I was ecstatic! Over the next few days I nursed him when he slept.

BACKGROUND NOTES

Breast refusal: What can cause it

The reasons your baby may suddenly refuse the breast aren't always easy to spot. But you can check some things routinely:

- *The baby's position.* Check that your baby is positioned well at the breast.

- *The position of the baby's tongue.* Some positions make it difficult for him to nurse.

- *Nipple confusion.* If your baby has been given a bottle previously, she may find it easier to bottle-feed than breastfeed. She may not remember how to suck at the breast.

- *Nipple shields.* Sometimes these are suggested for mothers with sore nipples. The baby can become used to nursing through the shield. She may refuse the breast without it.

- *Thrush.* A baby with thrush in his mouth can have a sore mouth. He may find it painful to nurse.

- *Strong let down.* If your let-down reflex acts quickly with a sudden gush of milk, your baby may choke as he tries to nurse. He may struggle and fight for breath and let go of the breast, coughing and sputtering. He may not want to nurse again.

- *Ear infection.* If your baby has had a cold or stuffy nose recently, she may have gotten an ear infection. This may cause pain when she tries to suck or swallow.

- *Reaction to something you have eaten.* Your baby may react to something you have eaten or drunk, or to a medication you have taken.

- *Change in taste of breast milk.* Some foods, drink or drugs can change the taste of your breast milk. Your baby may dislike the new taste. Mastitis or a blocked duct may also change the taste, sometimes only in the affected breast. Your milk may taste salty for a short time.

- *Change of smell.* Babies are very sensitive to smell. You may have changed your laundry soap or fabric softener. Or perhaps you are using a new deodorant, shampoo or hair-spray. Have you been given a new perfume recently? Your baby may object to any of these.

- *Menstruation.* Your breast milk may change a bit in taste or makeup when you have a period. Some babies do not like to nurse at this time, but nurse happily once your period is over.

- *Teething.* Your baby's gums and jaw may be tender when a tooth is growing. He may be reluctant to nurse.

- *A tough age.* Once your baby reaches four to six months, he may get distracted from the breast. He may also object to nursing in a noisy place.

FEEDING FILE

Breast refusal: What may help

- Try to stay calm. Your baby is not rejecting you. He needs you to help him through this tough time.

- Talk or sing to your baby. Comfort her with a soothing voice.

- Skin-to-skin contact is comforting. Cuddle him close, but do not try to breastfeed unless he clearly wants to.

- Try nursing when he is asleep or very sleepy.

- Change the way you hold your baby. Sit her up or lie down to nurse.

- Movement can be useful. Try rocking her or walking around to nurse. If you have a rocking chair, this may be soothing.

- Stimulate your let-down reflex before you offer the breast. If your baby gets an 'instant reward' for latching on, she may keep on nursing. This can help if your baby has become used to bottle-feeding, where she does not have to work for a let down. It may also help to express the first 'rush' of milk if you have a strong let-down reflex.

- Express your milk to keep your supply going until your baby wants to nurse again. You could feed the expressed milk from a cup until he is ready to go back to nursing.

- If you or your baby become upset while you are trying to get her to nurse, stop and try again later. Fighting with her will only make things worse.

- If your baby has become 'attached' to the nipple shield, try cutting the tip away. Cut away a bit more each day until you can nurse without it.

- Be patient. Be gentle. But don't give up!

(He still went wild if I tried when he was awake.) Then he began to open his eyes while he was nursing. At first he pulled away and cried and I would comfort him. But one day he opened his eyes and kept nursing happily. This whole thing took about two weeks."

Biting Babies

When your baby's teeth begin to come in, you may worry that your baby will bite you when he is nursing. In fact, most babies get their teeth and continue to nurse. Your baby needs to push his tongue out over his lower teeth when he is nursing. The "danger" time is often when he has finished nursing and wants to "play" at the breast. As he gets older, this playfulness may include a "nip" at the nipple as he lets go of the suction. Often a firm "No!" is enough to keep him from repeating the game.

Patti's first baby bit her once: *"I said, 'No!' loudly and firmly and removed him. He never bit again. My second bit me a few times, usually after cutting a new tooth. She made tiny square holes in my skin that were really painful. But once she got used to the new tooth (three to six days) we were back to normal."*

You may find a link between your baby biting you and something else, such as your period starting or something you ate or drank. This problem doesn't last long and may solve itself, as it did for Debbie: *"When my daughter was exactly a year old, she started biting me at every feeding (about three a day at the time). She would have her feeding, then, when she was done, she would get her teeth around my nipple and pull. She had never done it before and she stopped after a week. Then I realized I'd just had my first period. She had started biting me the day before the period began. She bit me again a couple of times when I had my next period and never did it again."*

Relactation

Breast milk is such a flexible resource. You can change your mind and begin to breastfeed again even if you have started giving bottles or have stopped breastfeeding completely. You can make this decision at any time after you have had a baby. It will be easier if you start again within a few weeks of your baby's birth. It is even possible to produce milk when you have not given birth. But in this case, you may find it harder to stimulate a full supply for your baby. Jenny managed to make the change from bottle to breast: *"I couldn't breastfeed. It hurt, and part of me was convinced that if Michele really was OK she'd have been able to nurse easily. Anyway, Michele drank well from a bottle. I knew she was sucking properly as I could see the milk go down. I began to regret not nursing her. On our first night at home she screamed while my husband warmed her bottle. In the hospital a bottle had been in the room when I needed it.*

"I didn't really think there was anything I could do. But I phoned a breastfeeding counselor to ask her advice. She told me it was possible. She advised me to try nursing Michele at frequent intervals. At first, she said, I'd need to supplement with formula until my milk supply got going again. I started trying that day. It wasn't easy. Michele was cheerful but a little confused. I was having the same problems I'd had the first night in the hospital. After a while I got her latched on.

FEEDING FILE

Biting Babies

When your baby might bite

- **Teething.** Teething babies like to chew. Give her something cool to chew on before nursing. If you use a teething gel, make sure you don't numb your baby's tongue. This can make it hard for her to latch on.

- **Slow let down.** Sometimes, your baby may want your milk to start flowing more quickly than your let down allows. She may bite to "speed things up." Check your baby's position. She will not nurse well if she is not latched on well. Try using warmth before nursing to help you relax and to speed up your let down.

- **Attention-seeking.** Your baby may want more of your attention than you are giving him when he is nursing, especially if he is older. Try giving him your complete attention. Talk to him and look into his eyes.

- **Distraction or lack of interest.** If you try to nurse your baby when she does not really want to, she may bite you when you try to get her to latch on. If something distracts her when she is nursing, she may bite as she turns to look at whatever has caught her interest. She may hold on to the nipple with her teeth. You may need to nurse in a quiet place for a while.

- **End of a feeding.** When your baby comes to the end of a feeding, she may bite as she lets go of your nipple. You may be able to watch for this. See if her jaw tightens before she bites down. Try to release the suction gently so she has to let go properly.

If your baby bites

- You may react strongly the first time your baby bites. You may scream or shout out and startle your baby. This may be enough to prevent her from biting again.

- He will not understand your distress. He may get scared by your sudden reaction and may refuse to nurse again. Try to stay calm.

- Try not to pull her off the breast while she is biting down. This will cause more damage. Slip your little finger into the corner of her mouth to release your nipple.

- Say "No!" firmly and stop nursing.

- If she persists, try seating her on the floor for a short time right after she bites. Most babies dislike being away from you like this. She may connect it with biting.

- If your nipples become sore, try the advice in chapter 8 for soothing sore nipples.

- Remember your baby does not know she is hurting you. She does not mean you any harm.

- Show your baby how happy you are when she nurses and does not bite you.

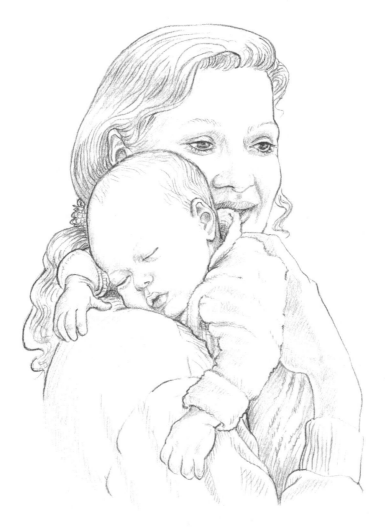

"It was hard. Michele lost a lot of weight at first. After her first breast-feeding, she refused formula milk totally! I still worried that Michele was getting 'enough' because I couldn't see milk disappear from a bottle. With help and support we got through the problems. Michele was fully breastfed from then on for 18 weeks. We kept nursing until she was eight months old."

Jenny was able to breastfeed completely again within a short time. Her supply was still fairly good. If you want to start again after a longer interval, you may need extra help. A breast pump can be helpful, to express

---

FEEDING FILE

Starting again: What may help

- Think positive. Your milk supply can be built up again. It is even possible to make milk when you have not given birth. Some mothers nurse their adopted babies.

- Breastfeed your baby before giving a bottle.

- Use any of the advice in chapter 4 to increase your milk supply and cut out extra bottles.

- A breast pump may help increase your supply. See chapter 11 for more about using a pump.

- Contact a breastfeeding counselor or your local La Leche League group for support and information.

---

milk and to stimulate your breasts between feedings. There is also a useful device called a "nursing supplementer," which Stephanie found was helpful: *"The breastfeeding counselor brought over a nursing supplementer. The baby sucks formula from a small tube taped to the nipple. This stimulates milk production. I started using it the next day. By the end of that week (Darryl was six weeks old), my breasts were much larger. I could express small spurts of milk. It was enough to prove it was working. I felt so much better trying it a second time.*

"At first, nursing had seemed so hard. Bottle-feeding seemed like a good solution. Now I feel great. It's been only three days since he wouldn't nurse at all, and now I can supply all his milk. And he's so eager to take it. I'm so glad I made the effort to try again. But it wasn't easy, especially finding the right people to give advice. Darryl is a happy baby now. We did it despite everything."

Using a nursing supplementer will stimulate milk production.

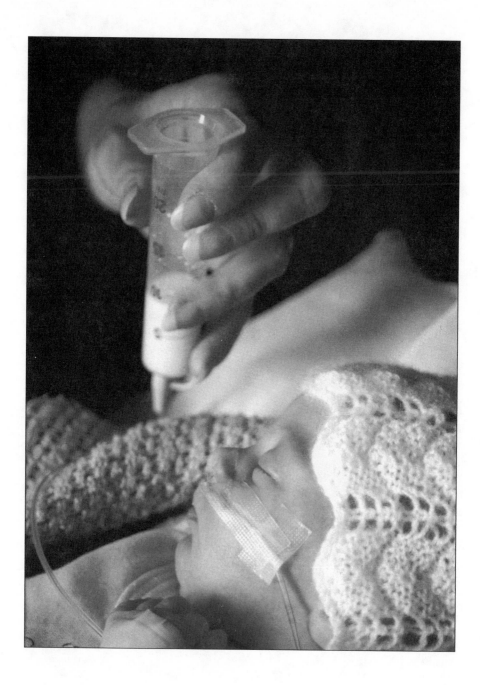

CHAPTER 10 *Breastfeeding in Special Circumstances*

Babies with Special Needs

Some babies have special needs that can affect breastfeeding. If your baby is premature, ill, or has a disability, it may take some effort to establish breastfeeding. Sometimes your baby may be unable to nurse from the breast for a short time. You may need help to establish and maintain a supply of expressed milk, which can be given to the baby by bottle, tube or cup.

Premature Babies

In 1990, 13% of babies born were admitted to neonatal intensive care units (NICUs). The Infant Feeding survey[1] showed that mothers of low-birthweight babies (babies less than 5-$\frac{1}{2}$ pounds) are less likely to breastfeed. Even if you begin, the lower the baby's weight at birth, the more likely you are to stop breastfeeding. There are many reasons for this. It is not easy to be in the hospital with your baby in the intensive-care unit. For premature babies, breast milk is extremely important. Much research has been done on the benefits of breast milk for these tiny babies.[55] But the hospital staff may not focus on this with you. They may be more anxious to put weight on the baby quickly.

Vanessa's son, Tony, was to stay in the intensive care unit for five weeks. She used the pump every three hours for much of that time: *"I was even more intent on breastfeeding Tony because I felt it was the only thing I could do for him. But I produced very little milk. Soon Tony's need for nutrition overtook my supply. Formula milk had to be given, first by tube through the nose, then by bottle."*

BACKGROUND NOTES

Milk for premature babies

Breast milk is important to premature babies. Studies have shown that giving premature babies their mother's breast milk reduces the chances of illness or death a great deal.[56] The best growth and development of the brain depends on the baby receiving essential fatty acids through breast milk,[18] as do the baby's eyes.[70]

The protective effect of breast milk is even more important in premature babies. *Necrotizing enterocolitis* (NEC) is a rare but very serious disease seen in premature babies. It is very rare for a baby given breast milk to get NEC.[73] Babies fed formula alone have a 6 to 10 times greater risk of getting this disease.[56]

But it's not easy to establish a milk supply when the baby may be too weak to suck at the breast. Some premature babies may be strong enough to nurse. Many will become exhausted if they try it. Others may not have developed a sucking reflex.

In these cases, a fine nasogastric tube is passed into the baby's stomach through the nose. Milk is fed through the tube. Breastfeeding is then begun slowly, as the baby grows stronger and her muscle tone improves enough to nurse.

Kelly's first child was in intensive care at first for about four days. But she was determined to nurse him: *"People kept saying: 'Don't worry, it'll come. We'll tube-feed him for now.' But I knew it was most important to put him to the breast whenever I could and he showed interest. He was on medications, too. People made me feel it was silly to try. But my gut feeling was to put him near me. Let him smell my breast. Let him feel me near him. And give him the chance to root (and me to bond with him, I suppose). And suddenly one night, despite being on drugs, he did begin to suck."*

The birth of a premature baby is often a time of crisis. It is a very emotional time. There may be concern for the baby's life. You may not be given the chance to nurse your baby in the delivery room. You may hardly see your baby before she is whisked away to intensive care. Then you are moved to a maternity ward. You may feel strange being there without a baby, next to new mothers with their babies. When you do see your baby in the incubator, she may be connected to several machines. One of the best things you can do for your new baby at this time is to begin to express your milk. Electric breast pumps are large, ugly and often housed in less-than-ideal places. It's hard to learn to use this machine and to learn how to produce milk at such a time. New mothers need a lot of support and encouragement, especially in the first few days. At first, a lot of effort seems to produce very little milk. A thoughtless comment or passing remark can cause hurt feelings and make some mothers want to give up. But a word of praise or encouragement will do wonders.

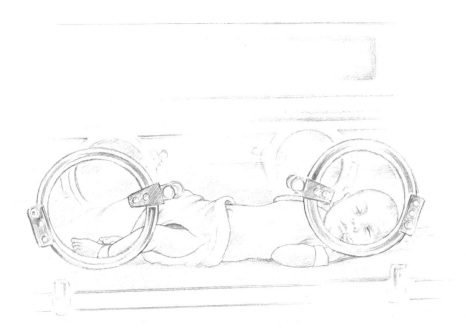

At 30 weeks' gestation, Rhonda had a second large blood loss and was whisked off to the labor ward: *"I was dilating quickly. But Karen was breech. I was told that a Cesarean was safer for her since she was so premature. When I woke up, Dean told me that we had a daughter in intensive care and first reports were good. It didn't take me long to fully come to. After the usual cleanup, I was wheeled up to see Karen. She was 3 lb. 6 oz. and tiny. She was on monitors and on a respirator. But she was ours and a healthy color. The next day, the nurse brought in a huge pump. We started the process of getting my milk supply going. I was determined to produce all that Karen required. For the time being, that was all I could do."*

Clare's son, Chris, was born five weeks too soon, before he got his sucking reflex: *"All day I kept asking about expressing. I was constantly told there was plenty of time for that later. Chris was born at 9 a.m. Finally, at about 9 p.m., they got someone to show me how to use the breast pump. A male nurse showed me how to use the machine. He showed me how to wash out all the parts, how to sterilize them, rinse them, and how to store and label the milk.*

FEEDING FILE

Starting a supply of breast milk

- Starting to breastfeed when the baby cannot suck at the breast is not easy. But it is possible.

- The most common method is to use an electric breast pump. Pumping needs to be started as soon as possible after birth. You may not be in any condition to think clearly about this at first. Often it is 24 to 48 hours before anyone has time to suggest using a pump.

- Most mothers do not let down well with the breast pump. The pump is a hard, cold machine. It gives you none of the stimulus that your warm, living baby does. You need a good pro-lactin response for your body to start milk production. This lack of prolactin response may be the reason some mothers produce a low volume of milk that is hard to sustain.[57,58]

- There are ways to improve the response. Some experts suggest massaging the breasts before beginning to express.[59] This will improve the supply of blood to the breasts, and stimulate the nipples. It mimicks the skin-to-skin contact you have with your baby.

- Stimulation will also induce a response from the other important breastfeeding hormone, oxytocin. This causes the let-down reflex.

- Instead of using a breast pump, express milk by hand. It's not hard to do. Once you have learned how, hand expressing works as well, or better, than using a pump. The fat content of hand-expressed breast milk may even be higher than that of pumped milk.[58]

- Whichever method you use, start early and express regularly. The breasts need to have milk removed frequently in order to keep the supply-and-demand cycle going.

- The rule, "the more milk is removed, the more will be produced," holds as true for expressing as it does for breastfeeding. Many mothers do not express their milk often enough to keep their supply going. Six to 8 times in 24 hours is the *minimum* requirement. This includes one night-time session, when prolactin levels are at their highest.[60]

- Premature babies only need a small amount of milk at one time. Express the foremilk into one container. Then express the rest of the milk for the baby to use right away. The foremilk can be used to "fill him up." In this way, the milk is likely to contain more fat, and therefore more calories. This will help the premature baby grow quickly. One expert suggests setting aside the first 25ml (a little less than 1 ounce).[59]

- Once the milk is expressed, it can be fed to the baby through the naso-gastric tube.

- Some neonatal intensive care units now use special plastic cups to feed babies who cannot nurse at the breast from birth, but whose mothers wish to breastfeed when they can. The cup is used instead of tube or bottle-feeding because it prevents babies from becoming confused between the different techniques of bottle- and breastfeeding.

FEEDING FILE (continued)

- One hospital tried a "preterm infant feeding protocol" for mothers with newborn babies admitted to the unit who wished to breastfeed. This involved massage, hand expression and frequent expression of milk, using tube or cup feeding until the babies were able to go to the breast. Using this protocol, the unit's breast-feeding success rate went up impressively, from 1% to 58%.[59]

- As soon as the premature baby shows any sign of being ready to suck, she should be put to the breast.

- Some hospitals prefer babies to move from tube-feeding to bottle-feeding and then to the breast. Others will allow the baby to go straight to the breast. It is often thought that bottle-feeding is "easier" than breastfeeding, but there is evidence that this may not be the case.[61]

"During this unpleasant experience, other mothers were waltzing into the same room. They took disposable bottles of sterilized, made-up formula, screwed on a disposable-ready sterilized nipple, and walked out full of the joys of spring. Meanwhile I sat there, huge sore boobs attached to an ugly machine straight out of a horror movie. It hurt. It was embarrassing. And I produced no milk at all. My baby was in intensive care being fed formula through a nose tube by a nurse. I really

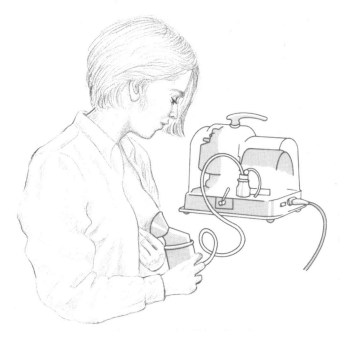

wanted someone to say: 'Good for you. You're doing the right thing for your baby. I know it hurts now but it will get easier. And you'll produce lots of milk and all will be well.' I said it to myself instead.

"*Three days later, through teeth-gritting pain and bleeding nipples, I produced one teaspoonful of colostrum. I was elated. This was greeted by a passing nurse with, 'That's no good. You need lots more than that.'*

"*In the neonatal intensive care unit, my breastmilk was treated more positively. It was given to Chris as part of his next feeding. I was delighted. They had more time in intensive care. They helped me put Chris to the breast before each tubefeeding. He couldn't really do it at all.*"

To begin with, many premature babies are fed by a tube that is passed through the nose into the stomach—*a nasogastric tube.* Once you are able to express colostrum, then breast milk, the fluids can be fed to your baby through the tube. Very tiny babies do not need much food. A teaspoonful of colostrum can be a whole feeding for a very small baby. Depending on the baby's condition, she may be able to breast-feed at a later stage.

As soon as the baby shows any desire to suck, you can help her to go to the breast. Even if she does not nurse for very long, or very well, the close skin contact with your breast will stimulate your milk supply. Some mothers feel that the baby does not 'belong' to them. The baby is surrounded by machines and cared for by intensive-care staff. You may feel that you need to "ask permission" to put your baby to the breast.

Suzanne was taught by a nurse to tube-feed her twins next to her breast. Then she gradually allowed them to suck at the same time, until their reflex was strong enough to remove the tube: "*Then I began trying to*

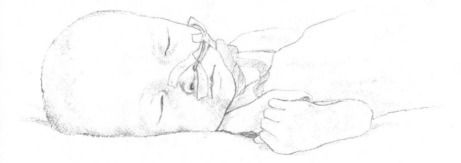

nurse them both at once. I stayed there day and night for a few days to
see if I could cope. Those were desperate days. I was desperate to take
them home. But I worried that they weren't getting enough. I didn't do
much else but nurse day and night."*

Every time Anna visited the intensive care unit, two floors up, she put
her baby to the breast: *"The nurses tried to be helpful but weren't,
really. They wanted to give her a measured amount of milk. This was
expressed breast milk (some of it mine) for the first four days. Then the
milk bank was low. So as the healthiest baby on the unit, my baby had
to go on formula. I was getting out a tiny amount with the pump. Using
the pump hurt. I was in pain from my C-section and the after-pains,
too. I asked for her nasogastric tube to be left in longer and that she not
be given bottles. I hoped that I would begin nursing at the breast before
she got too used to the bottle nipple."*

Susan found that expressing was vital: *"Karen was breastfeeding once
a day by week two. It increased slowly. She was nursing with me all day
and on bottles of expressed milk at night until she was able to come
home in week seven. My supply was greater than her needs at this
stage—I had continued to express while nursing her during the day."*

A supportive NICU nurse helped Vanessa make contact with her premature son: *"After about 2-½ weeks, during a once-daily cuddle with
Tony, an intensive-care-unit nurse suggested I put him to my breast. It
was as if I needed permission to do this. The hospital had robbed me of
my motherhood. I wondered why I had not thought to do this before
now. I was thrilled at the prospect. My breasts would at long last come
into contact with the little mouth that needed me to feed it.*

*"I was lucky that the nurse was not too busy that day. She showed me
how I should position Tony at the breast. Once he was there, Tony didn't
exactly suck. (I was warned that he was still too weak to suck well.) But
he sniffed and played with the nipple in his mouth. It was the first time
I felt a let-down sensation. The nurse was great. She said things like,
'Isn't that wonderful? Look, he knows what to do! What a good little
boy!' I remember glowing with pride."*

Even having more than one premature baby can become less daunting
with help and support, as Donna describes: *"I tried breastfeeding the
babies when they were 10 days old. To my amazement they (all four
quads) managed to nurse a little, despite their tiny birth weights (rang-
ing from 3 to 4 pounds)."*

Many mothers of premature babies leave the hospital before their babies. This adds to the problems of expressing milk for the baby. Now it has to be brought to the hospital. Trips to and from the intensive care unit are stressful for a new mother. You may be able to rent or borrow an electric breast pump from the hospital.

To meet the baby's needs, pumping must be done at the same times a baby would nurse. This means you have to have a pump at home and at the hospital. You also must be able to store the expressed milk until it can be taken to the baby. Many mothers are able to sustain a milk supply with the pump. They breastfeed their babies during their visits to hospital. They often feel that it is the most important thing they can do for their premature baby. Nursing also helps to foster a bond between mother and baby.

Donna's babies stayed in the hospital for about a month. She rented an electric breast pump and traveled in with her expressed breast milk: *"After 10 days, the babies were mainly bottle-fed. They only had small feedings from me when I could manage it.*

"I use the breast pump, which has two cups, between six and 10 times a day, depending on how much help I have and how tired I am. It takes me about 15 minutes to express between 6 and 16 fluid ounces. The amount I can express depends on the time of day, the amount of fluid and food intake I've managed and again, how tired I am.

"Despite it being a boring task, and very tiring, I have kept using the breast pump. I know that the babies have had between a quarter and two-thirds of their feedings from me. I am convinced that it has been a big factor in the continued good health of our babies. It has also given me a few 15-minute breaks alone each day.

"Although a breast pump may be expensive to rent, it is a small price to pay for the priceless breast milk you can give your baby. It also saves on buying formula milk."

Once your baby is strong enough to nurse from the breast, it is best to do so at frequent intervals. Sometimes there may be a conflict between nursing in order to increase supply and keeping a record of the baby's intake, as Vanessa describes: *"When I tried to breastfeed during my hospital visits, it was a problem for the intensive-care-unit staff. They wanted to measure fluid intake to assess growth and development. They would ask me how much milk he had taken. How did I know?"*

You may find it hard to trust that your body is making enough milk for your baby, once you can no longer see the milk flowing into the pump. Very small babies may have trouble getting a good latch. Skilled help at this stage is vital.

Vanessa found that she could latch Tony on with a little help: *"As Tony progressed from intensive care to the the normal newborn nursery, we tried to master breastfeeding together. (We hoped to cut out the formula feedings.) Tony was still small and had trouble latching on. One nurse suggested a nipple shield. Another nurse expressed concern about using one. To prevent nipple-shield dependence, I would remove the shield as soon as the nipple was drawn out. Then Tony could latch on directly. I used this method for about five days. Tony and I kept nursing (along with bottle-feedings) until he was over nine months old."*

For some mothers, like Valarie, sadly, the struggle is just too great: *"I was encouraged to breastfeed (29-week-old, 2-½-pound baby). I used an electric pump while she was in the hospital. She had trouble learning to nurse, but managed after a while with a nipple shield. My milk supply never built up enough. I did everything I could to keep on breastfeeding. But she didn't gain weight for two weeks or more. At that point, I was advised to supplement but to breastfeed, too. This was the worst of all worlds, because she needed extra at every feeding. After five months, she began to refuse the breast and I gave up with relief."*

When the day comes to take your premature baby home, you may find you are not sure if you can cope without the support of the intensive care unit. You may have built good relationships with the staff. At home, visits with your pediatrician, although they may be more frequent to start with, are not the same as 'on the spot' help and advice. Sometimes it can seem as if your baby's doctor is not on the same wavelength. But sometimes she can help sustain you against those who doubt your ability to provide milk for your baby.

Rhonda relied on her husband and her pediatrician to give her the confidence she needed to carry on: *"During the first months at home, Karen nursed so often that I would hear comments from friends or family members to put her on a bottle: 'You couldn't possibly have any milk left.' Comments like these eroded my confidence. I needed a lot of encouragement to ignore them and believe in myself. Dean was great at this. And my pediatrician helped me through one bad time by suggesting that I think things over for a few days before making a decision.*

That helped put things in perspective. Looking back at Karen's first months, I think I encountered many events that new mothers do. But since Karen was older (by the calendar) when she came to these stages, I often became anxious. I worried it was a sign that things were not going normally."

Babies Who Are Ill or Have Special Needs

It is very upsetting to learn that your new baby may not be well. Unless you have breastfed before, it can be hard to think about starting to express at such a time.

The neonatal intensive care unit may not be close to the maternity ward. Some mothers, who may have just had a difficult birth, find they have the added stress of being apart from their baby. If the baby is not premature, and you're OK, you may be able to breastfeed sooner than with a premature baby. All the special benefits of breast milk will be even more important for a baby who has other challenges to face in his new life.

Sometimes, though, nursing may be restricted. Breastfeeding may be delayed until the baby's condition improves, as with Cindy's baby: *"After her birth, she did not want to nurse, which was very upsetting for me. Her sisters had nursed soon after birth. I had a bad feeling when she didn't want to. She kept changing color. Finally she was diagnosed as a 'grunting' baby (a baby with a breathing problem). An hour after she was born, she was whisked away to intensive care, where she spent six days. For the first four days, she was fed 100% by IV and was sur-rounded by wires and monitors. I was only allowed to touch her through the access holes in the incubator. My first visit to the nursery was really hard for me.*

"I wanted to start expressing as soon as possible. It was really good for me to be doing something to help. At four days, they started with tube feedings. Then, a day and a half later, I was told I could nurse her myself. She latched on as if she had been nursing from day one! It was a wonderful moment. The next 24 hours were frustrating. They kept test weighing, which I didn't think was too accurate. Each feeding was fol-lowed with a tubefeeding. She had to be fed every four hours. So when I showed up, she was still full and sleepy from her last feeding. She didn't take a lot and had to be fed with a tube as well. It went on like this.

"With support from the staff in my ward, I pushed the nursery staff to put her on demand feeding. Finally they agreed, but only if she stayed

with them. This meant taking a hike, because we were on opposite ends of the hospital! I was also still getting over my third C-section. But that was the furthest thing from my mind at that point. After only two feedings, she was allowed back with me at 10:30 p.m. one night. It felt like having her all over again!"

Celia thought everything was going well, but then her baby became ill: *"Rebecca was born at home in an ideal birth. Labor was four to five hours with no problems, no pain relief and a very serene setting. She was put to the breast right away and sucked away happily for over half an hour. I felt wonderful and on top of the world. She was born at 2:30 a.m., so we all dozed until morning. At 7 a.m., she started to get sick. We called the doctor. We were sent to the hospital and Rebecca was put in intensive care. I insisted on nursing her that day. By evening I was exhausted. They bottle-fed her in the night.*

"Rebecca was allowed out of intensive care the next day and I nursed her during the day. She started to get sick again that night and was put back into intensive care. Finally, they decided she had meningitis. All feeding stopped and she went on restricted fluids. That day my milk came in and my breasts were huge, hot and sore. I went on the electric pump and froze the expressed milk. I wondered if Rebecca would live to drink it. For the next two days, I pumped every four hours and built up a small collection of frozen milk. Then Rebecca got better, and she was sucking madly. The doctors said I could nurse her once a day. What bliss! She nursed so well and relaxed afterwards. I decided that if she lived I would breastfeed her, whatever the problems.

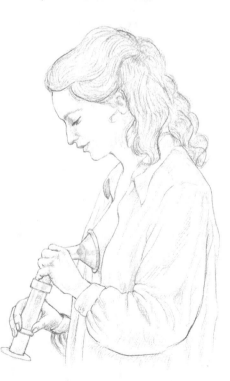

"For the next few days, I nursed her when I was allowed to. I pumped the rest of the time. Soon I was feeding her completely. Then I got sore, cracked and

BACKGROUND NOTES

Cleft lip and/or palate

Breastfeeding is likely to be harder for a baby with a cleft lip or palate. It can be harder for him to maintain the seal between mouth and breast that is required to create a good suck. Even if a baby with a severe cleft can't breastfeed, he will still benefit a great deal from being fed breast milk. Breast milk has immune-enhancing properties.

Babies with clefts are prone to ear infections, because of a higher chance of liquid filling the Eustachian tubes when the baby swallows. (Eustachian tubes lead from the back of the nose to the inner ear.) Breastfed babies with clefts have 75% fewer ear infections and infections of the upper respiratory tract than formula-fed babies. And because it is a natural body fluid, breast milk will not irritate mucous membranes if it ends up in the "wrong place."

Breastfeeding is an important factor in improving the strength of facial muscles. That will help the baby's face develop normally. It may also help normal speech develop, because of the effort involved in nursing. The tongue and gums get exercised in a very specific way.

The position of the cleft will determine the position the baby needs to be in to make a seal and start nursing. A cleft in the soft or hard palate can make it harder for a mother to position her baby at the breast so the breast will be stripped well of milk. The baby needs to be able to squeeze the nipple and breast tissue against the roof of his mouth, pressing on the collected milk. If the cleft is large, this may not be possible. Milk may also leak into the nasal passages, which can cause choking. A dental plate may be made to cover the cleft, which can help. Consult your dentist to find out more.

Breasts are soft and can mold to the required shape more easily than bottles with nipples. Sometimes the mother's thumb can cover any remaining gap between breast and mouth to enable the baby with a cleft lip to nurse well. Often babies with clefts swallow more air than other breastfed babies. They may need to be burped during a feeding.

Surgery

Treatment for a cleft lip or palate will begin in the first few months of life. Repairs to the lip are often done quite early. Repairs to the palate may be done at 6 months to 2 years of age. Surgeons differ in their opinions about when breastfeeding can begin again after a repair operation. There are several different ways to feed a baby who cannot breastfeed right after his operation. Most hospitals can give guidance about this.

Special guidance

About Face is a support and information organization concerned with facial differences. It also supports Cleft Parent Guilds, support groups of parents of children with a cleft lip or palate.

In the United States, call 1-800-225-FACE. E-mail: AbtFace@aol.com.

In Canada, call 1-800-665-FACE.

The **Cleft Palate Foundation** offers free information and referral services. Call 1-800-242-5338.

Write them at: 1218 Grandview Ave., Pittsburgh, PA 15211.

You can contact the **American Cleft Palate-Craniofacial Association** through this group.

bleeding nipples—terrible pain! Still, I was determined to give her the best. She needed any immunity I could give her in my breast milk. This thought kept me going.

"After 10 days, I had to go home and leave Rebecca in the hospital. I rented an electric pump to pump milk at night. I was able to get to the hospital by 7 a.m. I nursed her all day until 6 p.m. Then I pumped milk at night and at 1:30 in the morning to take in for her for the next night. The night nurses were great. They fed her with my expressed breast milk and used the frozen supplies when she needed more than I could supply. When the frozen supplies were used up, the supplemented the fresh expressed breast milk with formula.

"After 17 days in the hospital, Rebecca came home. I started nursing her all the time then. It was very, very hard. I got very sore."

Holly's baby Joe was diagnosed with "clicky hips" (hips that are dislocated). He was put into a splint. Although the splint was awkward, she thought it wouldn't cause a problem: *"Nursing from my left breast was fine. But for some unknown reason, he would not latch on to my right breast. I was told by the hospital nurse to hold him under my arm with his legs behind me. That worked, but it wasn't very comfortable. And it was harder to feed discreetly. Unless I was in my own house with pillows for him to lie on, the problems were getting worse. As he got heavier and his legs got longer, he was still in a frog position from the splint. I was getting a little upset. He was still nursing fine from the left. I kept putting him across me on the right but he still would not latch on. Nursing would last between an hour and an hour and a half. It seemed to be about every three hours. It was hard work.*

"Finally the cause was found. At his eight-week hip check, he was diagnosed as having a bad neck (torticollis). This is where the neck muscle is stretched and then contracts. His head constantly fell to the side. He started physical therapy right away. But by the time his neck problem was cured and his splint was off, he had put on very little weight. I was advised to supplement with bottle milk. By five months I had dried up completely."

For some mothers, like Mina, despite their desire, their baby's condition does not allow them to breastfeed: *"When my son was born prematurely, I wanted to breastfeed. I hadn't even bought a bottle or sterilizers! But he couldn't breastfeed or bottle-feed. He was born with a severe bilateral cleft lip and palate. The only way I could get milk inside him—with a struggle—was to spoon-feed."*

FEEDING FILE

Positions for feeding a baby with a cleft

Feeding may take much longer than normal. It pays to be patient and to experiment. A more upright position than normal is often better for the baby. This position helps prevent milk from leaking into the nasal passages. No matter what position you decide is best, keep your baby facing you. Keep his head and neck in line. Do not let him twist around, which would make it harder for him to swallow.

Straddle position

Seat your baby in your lap, facing you, with his legs on either side of your stomach. You may need to seat him on pillows to bring him up to the level of your breast. Then see where to position your nipple so that he can get the best latch. It may help to tilt the baby's head back a bit as he latches on. Then you are free to use your other hand to help the baby make a seal between his mouth and your breast, or simply to support his chin.

Football hold

The football hold described in chapter 7 can be changed to suit the baby's needs. Again, pillows may be needed to raise the baby up to the level of your breast. Position your baby so he is sitting up beside you, facing you, with his legs and feet under your arm. Support your baby with your arm, and his head gently in your hand. You may need to support your breast with your other hand to help the baby make a seal.

Preference for one side

Depending on the position of the cleft, some babies may have a strong preference for nursing in one position. Changing sides may not be easy. It may be better for you to keep the baby in his preferred position. Simply slide him across to the other breast. Or just nurse him from one breast.

Breastfeeding in a Children's Hospital

It can be hard for you as a breastfeeding mother if your baby needs admission to a children's hospital. The staff may lack training and time to help with breastfeeding. Or the schedule does not support breastfeeding. You can't be certain that anyone in a children's hospital will know or be up-to-date about breastfeeding.

At five weeks, Rose's baby had a bad case of croup. They were admitted to the local hospital: *"He made an amazing noise as he coughed. He screamed at the same time so the doctor couldn't hear a thing through her stethescope when she tried to examine him. I wanted to let him nurse to calm him down. But the look I got from the nurse will always stay with me. As soon as the exam was over, she sent a janitor in to us with*

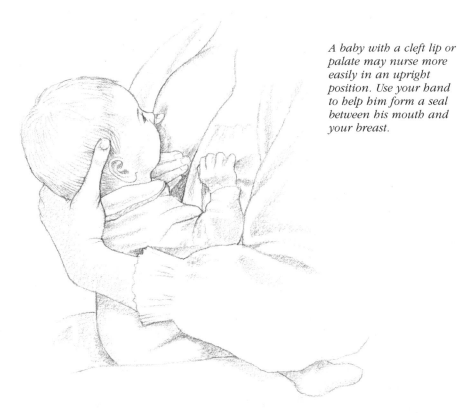

A baby with a cleft lip or palate may nurse more easily in an upright position. Use your hand to help him form a seal between his mouth and your breast.

screens. Then she read me the riot act about nursing behind these in case someone walked through the ward and saw me nursing a baby! I felt more alone than ever.

"The maternity unit in the hospital had an amazing lady known as the lactation nurse. She promoted breastfeeding on the maternity wards. They called for her to watch me nurse and prove that I could do it. I felt, as she watched, that my milk flow was being measured. But it was a relief to have her confirm my feeling as to the amount he was taking, even if she did talk about my droopy breasts!

"One of the younger doctors worried that he had no record of the amount that the baby was getting. One suggested that they needed an IV just because he was breastfed, in case he became dehydrated. The nursing staff insisted we fill in a chart listing how long he nursed. They didn't think my estimate of how much he was taking might be useful. I *began to wish that my breasts had lines like a measuring cup. I was criticized constantly by the nursing staff for nursing him on demand. I felt that if he had enough strength to try to nurse and breathe, then I wanted him to get some nourishment. But all the other children on the ward were fed every four hours. I was lucky to have my mom's support. She had been a midwife in the days when not to breastfeed a baby was so abnormal that it was recorded in a midwife's log.*

"As Patrick began to get better, the doctors began to really get on my case about nursing on demand. I was told that nursing more often than every four hours tired the mother and this deprived the rest of my family. As the mother of a less than 2-year-old and a baby who could rarely sleep more than an hour before his breathing trouble woke him, I told them I was pleased to be able to sit down every couple of hours, have a drink, read to my toddler and nurse my baby."

Admission to a children's hospital can be even harder if facilities for mothers are also limited. Finding enough food for a breastfeeding mother may be a problem. Lena felt that her needs were not considered at all: *"My daughter was transferred to a children's hospital at birth. I chose to go with her to breastfeed and closely follow her progress. Care is focused on the babies. But newly delivered mothers need care too, especially at times like this. The lack of a bed was the worst thing. Taking a nap or resting during the day was impossible. I had a folding bed at night in a small closet. Postnatal exercises were hard to do. I had little privacy for exams. Facilities were poor. The restrooms were in a different wing. The cafeteria was far away. And there was one filthy shower. There was no breastfeeding advice or support—the staff had no experience or training. Nurses with children themselves were more helpful. But many younger nurses didn't know what to do with a tearful mom who had problems breastfeeding."*

Babies with special needs who are able to nurse at the breast will gain comfort from the contact, besides the benefit of breast milk.

Breastfeeding may also help you bond with your baby. Supplying milk for your baby may be the only thing you can do to help the medical staff care for him. Roseanne needed to feel close to her son. His condition was serious: *"Breastfeeding my baby with his uncertain diagnosis was the best thing for both of us. We remained close and untouched by what seemed to be disastrous events. Even when his echocardiogram (ultrasound of the heart) confirmed that our second son had a congenital*

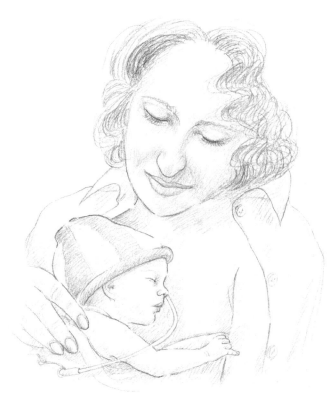

large-heart defect (40% of children with Down syndrome have it), I still wanted to nurse him. The doctors said he would not gain weight quickly and could need extra feedings. We had to bring him back for weight checks and blood tests for some time after his discharge from the hospital. By the time the Down syndrome had been confirmed we were convinced, though we still prayed it wouldn't be true. Our start together was a bumpy one. But breastfeeding was never a problem. It was the one joy I had planned for that no one could take away!"

When Gail's second son Phillip was only two days old, he was found to be suffering from a major heart defect and was admitted to the hospital. He had a minor operation that night to stabilize his condition. Then he had to wait a week before the open-heart surgery to fix the problem: *"I had breastfed my older son for almost a year. I was anxious to do the same for Phillip. It was important for me, when so much depended on the skills of the surgeons and medical staff, to feel that there was at least one thing I could do to give him the best possible chance of coming through the operation.*

"Luckily, the hospital was able to give me a room in the same building as the children's ward. The nursing staff would call me down for nighttime feedings. Phillip nursed so well that he'd regained his birthweight after only five days.

"A couple of days before the operations, I started to practice expressing milk with an electric pump, in a tiny room close to the ward. I froze the milk in small amounts for use later. During the time Phillip was in intensive care, I expressed three times a day. I produced about 6 ounces at each session.

"After the first day in intensive care, Phillip was allowed to receive increasing amounts of my expressed milk through a nasogastric tube. Once again, it felt very good to know that I was doing my share to help his recovery. On the evening of the second day after the operation, Phillip was taken off the respirator. I was able to give him a small breastfeeding—an experience I felt we'd both been missing.

"Over the next couple of days, because Phillip's fluid intake still had to be limited, I breastfed him 'restrictively.' He was not encouraged to nurse, nor to return to the breast if he came off. After that, we were able to return to normal demand nursing."

Sometimes you may find that, when an older baby who is still breastfeeding falls ill, keeping up your supply becomes a lifeline for you. When Roseanne's son, Tom, was 11 months old, she suffered a frightening experience: *"Tom had a bad cold. He had been very needy, wanting to be at the breast all the time. I was very sore and gave him to Dad. He finally fell asleep. When he woke up, he was crying and upset. I cleared his nose and put him on my shoulder to take him downstairs to nurse. But when I placed him across my lap I noticed he was staring with both eyes towards the left. He could not suck at my breast. He could not move his right arm or leg. He had had a stroke.*

"After seven days on a respirator, and 10 days in the intensive care unit, the doctors didn't know if he would live. My milk supply was almost gone. Although I was hearing that there may be no baby to give my milk to, I felt strongly it was the bond that kept us united. I arranged to use an electric pump. I began with half an ounce and built up to three or four ounces. It helped keep me going somehow. It moved my thoughts from pity to hope. Once Tom came off the respirator and tube-feedings were begun, he was given my milk, supplemented with soy milk. Oh, the joy when Tom was released to the children's ward and he turned to breastfeed! I had not been sure that it would ever happen! I was so glad that I had not given up totally."

Mothers with Special Needs

If you are disabled or become ill, you may need special help with breastfeeding. Sometimes your caregivers may feel that breastfeeding will only add to the strain on your system. But you may want to keep on breastfeeding. Sensitive caregivers will help you come to terms with your loss if you have to stop. In many cases, with understanding and treatment, breastfeeding can continue.

Sylvia had a brain operation for an aneurysm (a ballooned and weakened blood vessel). As a result, she lost some nerve function and developed weakness on her right side: *"I have very little use of my right arm, and it's hard to walk. It's a little better when I wear an electronic stimulator. My son was two when it happened. Since then I have had a daughter. Breastfeeding my son was a lovely experience and I wanted to breastfeed my daughter. The benefits of breastfeeding are all there, but more so in my case. It meant that the problems of making and giving a bottle with one hand were gone.*

"Of course, I expected more problems nursing my daughter than I had with my son. But I found that they could all be dealt with. For example, I was able to manage holding the baby while she nursed by using pillows. I was able to buy a V-shaped pillow that was ideal and provided secure support. Having breastfed before my loss of arm and leg function, I knew that most of the problems I had were what any mother would be faced with, whether disabled or not."

Not only was Helen's son diagnosed as allergic to formula milk, but he also had a medical problem. Breastfeeding, or any type of feeding, became harder. And then Helen learned she was ill: *"I suddenly started losing dramatic amounts of weight (without trying). I was finally reserred to a specialist. I was diagnosed as having a condition often referred to as gluten allergy (though it is not really an allergy). My system couldn't absorb vitamins and minerals properly. So I had a fairly small baby and too few resources to establish a good milk supply. As soon as I started a gluten-free diet, I began to feel better. Finally I had a reason for my failure to breastfeed.*

"Now I'm considered perfectly healthy. (I'm glad to say my son is, too!) I still regret not being able to give my son the very best start in life. But I can be happy that I did what I could at the time. I am told that if I follow a strict diet, I should be able to fully breastfeed any other children I might have."

A sudden illness can disrupt breastfeeding. If your milk supply is well established, it doesn't mean the end of breastfeeding, though. If you are admitted to a hospital, you should be able to take your fully breast-fed baby with you. Norma found that frequent breastfeeding helped her supply come back: *"When Sarah was about three months old, I caught a horrible stomach bug, which meant I didn't eat for several days. I couldn't keep down water for two days. My doctor poked my breasts and laughed, 'Ha! Empty! Get a can of formula, your breast-feeding days are over!' I ignored her advice and let Sarah nurse often. I did give her a little boiled water from a spoon too because I was wor-ried that she'd dehydrate. My milk soon returned when I could keep water down."*

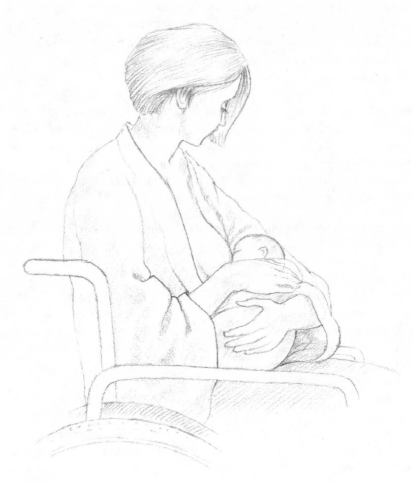

Breastfeeding may have practical advantages for you.

Janet suffers from chronic asthma: *"Pregnancy was good for my asthma. (But I was still on high doses of inhaled steroids and had to have one course of steroid tablets.) Now my asthma is worse again. Besides helping protect Emma from asthma and eczema, breastfeeding has been helpful to me. The ease, especially at night, is a real bonus. I am often breathless at night when I nurse her. But all I have to do is take a few puffs of my inhaler and I can nurse her right away. I make life even easier for myself by having Emma sleep in bed with me so I don't even have to get up.*

> ## BACKGROUND NOTES
>
> ### Able Parents
>
> Parents with a disability can contact their local Public Health Department (in the United States) or Ministry of Health (in Canada) for referral and support.
>
> **Suggested reading:**
>
> *The Baby Challenge: A handbook on pregnancy for women with a physical disability.* M.J. Campion. London: Tavistock/Routledge, 1990.
>
> *Mother to be: A guide to pregnancy and birth for women with disabilities.* J. Rogers and M. Matsumura. New York: Demos, 1991.

"The weight of the baby on my chest can be a problem, but I can support her on a pillow on my lap. That really reduces the pressure on my chest. (I wanted to nurse her lying down, but that has not been possible. I cannot breathe well lying on my side.) Sometimes when I cough I throw Emma off my breast. This can give me a sore nipple. But Emma seems to take it in her stride and the soreness doesn't last long. Bottle-feeding at night would be hard, because I would have to get up and do things.

"The other advantage of breastfeeding is that the prolactin hormone you produce when nursing relaxes you. That's always a bonus for an asthmatic, because you need less oxygen when you are relaxed. Tension can make the wheezing worse. And I don't need to carry the bottle-feeding junk around, like sterile water, powder and bottles. The less I need to carry the better, because I just cannot carry things when I am breathless."

Sometimes it takes time and cleverness to find the best solution to practical problems.

Libby has had ME (myalgic encephalomyelitis) for nearly 11 years. During that time, she has had two babies and has breastfed both. ME affects the muscles and brain. Her main symptoms are fatigue, muscle pain and weakness, memory problems and feeling really cold: *"With the first baby, it was hard to get comfortable. The baby felt heavy. It was a strain. And night feedings meant I got very cold. With the second, I did better in every respect. (But the second pregnancy made my ME much worse.) This time, though, I knew how to breastfeed. I found ways to handle the ME problems. I lay on the bed with the baby's weight on my body. (I'd tried to sit up with the first one.) That solved the weight and muscle problems. I had the baby by my side at night. (The first one had been in a separate room.) This way neither of us became cold."*

Isla's right hand is affected by cerebral palsy: *"I can't move my fingers on that hand. This caused problems when breastfeeding. So my one-day-old baby son and I had to try different positions and pillows until we found a way that suited us. It was only a small problem. But it seemed like a big one at the time. I did feel very lonely because the hospital nurses either couldn't understand the problem or didn't have time to help me solve it. I wanted to find an answer quickly, not weeks after giving birth. I had my daughter when my son was less than two years old, so I had my hands full. I really believe that you can find an answer if you are a little creative."*

Renée was sent to bed with a back problem for six weeks, when her son Brian was two weeks old: *"I'd nursed Brian lying down before, in the hospital and at home. But now I had two slipped discs and it all got pretty tricky fast! Nursing involved lying on my side while getting Brian in position and latched on with one hand. I had to hold a breast shield in the cup of my nursing bra with the other. (Nursing bras are made to support the other breast when the owner sits up, not when she is on her side). When he'd finished the first side, I'd have to go through some very tricky moves to turn me and him over. I'd fix the drip-spotted towel we were lying on. And we'd start the whole thing again on side two. Still, it was really worth it: I couldn't do anything else for Brian at this time, or for myself. This seemed to be the single part of motherhood at which I excelled. I really wanted to hang on to it."*

Extra help with household tasks and caring for other children may be vital for you if you need extra rest to maintain your milk supply. If this doesn't happen, you may feel as Cheryl did: *"The main problem this time was that I was so tired. I couldn't keep up with the demand and I couldn't rest enough to improve it. I had an older child to consider. I didn't have the energy to keep nursing my baby more often because it left little or no time for rest or sleep."*

The psychological benefits of breastfeeding are also important. Janie explains why it is important to her: *"Because of my disability (I have multiple sclerosis and use a wheelchair when I go out), I feel I have to prove I can manage better than everyone else just so people don't think I'm helpless. I think breastfeeding Hannah helped in that respect. People could see she was really my baby. And she was growing and thriving because of the milk I was giving her."*

Should you suffer from postpartum depression, you may find, as these mothers did, that breastfeeding is an important way to build your self-confidence at a time when you may be feeling low.

"Despite suffering from postpartum depression after the birth of my first baby, I found great comfort in being able to breastfeed. I did not feel that my mothering skills were very good. But at least my growing baby helped me see that I was taking care of at least one part of motherhood."

"My main symptom was extreme tiredness. It was almost impossible to get up and get dressed, let alone do housework or shop. I don't think I would ever have managed to fix bottles. Lying in bed nursing Sara was about all I could manage."

Breastfeeding after Breast Surgery

If you have had any kind of breast surgery before having children, you may wonder, like Laurie, whether you will be able to breastfeed: *"When I was 19, I had a benign lump removed from my right breast. At the time, I only worried whether the lump was malignant or not. But at 26, I was expecting our first baby. I really wanted to breastfeed. I began to wonder if I would have any problems due to my rigid scar.*

"Ruth was born and nursed well from both sides. By five or six months she was on to puréed food and gave up nursing from the right breast. Since I had dropped one feeding and she slept through the night, I figured I had less milk. I kept nursing her from the left side until she was 11 months.

"When Libby, our second daughter, was born, she gave up on the right breast after only a few weeks. But with the advice that 'twins manage on one' ringing in my ears, I kept nursing her until 11 months, just from the one side."

Your ability to breastfeed may depend on the surgery you have had done and how long ago it was performed. A simple 'lumpectomy,' as

Laurie describes, is not likely to damage the breast enough to prevent all milk production. She found that the breast that had undergone surgery did not seem to produce as much milk. But this is not always the case. Your surgeon may be the best person with whom to discuss your chances of success. He should be able to tell you if he had to cut through any milk ducts.

If you can still feel sensation in your nipples, breastfeeding will probably be easier for you. It means that you do not have much damage to your nerves. You may feel that, even if you can't produce all the milk your baby needs, it will be worth breastfeeding anyway. You could talk through your feelings about this with a breastfeeding counselor.

If you have had cosmetic surgery—augmentation or reduction—you may still be able to breastfeed. Again, this will depend on how much damage was done to the structure of the ducts during the operation. Silicone bags inserted behind the breast tissue, to enlarge the breasts, are less likely to interfere with breastfeeding. But you may feel worse at first when your milk comes in.

A reduction operation may cause more problems if the nipple has been moved. This procedure is likely to have involved cutting the ducts. Sometimes the ducts will knit together again, but this cannot be predicted. Again, your surgeon will be the best person to give you advice. If only one breast has had surgery, you will be able to breastfeed from the other.

The benefits of breastfeeding are greater for mothers and babies with special needs than for others. For the babies, breastfeeding offers comfort and health benefits. For you, there are practical advantages and the morale boost that successful breastfeeding brings. Both you and your baby need the best possible help and support to establish breastfeeding, taking account of your own circumstances and needs.

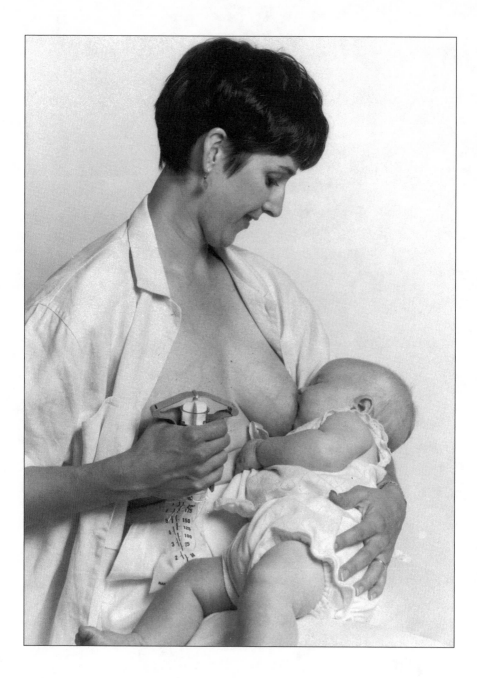

CHAPTER 11 *Breastfeeding and Returning to Work*

It has become common for women to return to paid work within a few months of the birth of their baby. You may have financial pressures to return to work, or concerns about career progress if you are away for long. Or it may be your choice. Those who have more than basic maternity pay and leave may not return to work so soon. But many mothers return after a 12 weeks' maternity leave or sooner, depending on their circumstances.

There is little current information about the effect of going back to work on breastfeeding. Does an early return to work prevent mothers from starting to breastfeed? Does it affect how long they nurse? A study of mothers in 1990 found that mothers of first babies who were working tended to be more likely to breastfeed than those who were not working. It found no evidence that returning to work shortened the length of time a mother breastfed.[1] Whether such findings will remain true as more mothers of young babies go back to work remains to be seen.

Natalie made arrangements at work that helped her be with her baby as long as possible: *"I took the maximum maternity leave from work (paid and unpaid). Then I arranged with my employer to take all the vacation time I'd saved at the rate of 2-½ days a week. This gave me seven months off and up to three months of part-time work, before going back full time. Because of this long maternity leave, I always planned to breastfeed Esther. I continued with a morning and evening feeding as long as she wanted it."*

For Mandy, who returned to work sooner, the choice was harder: *"I felt pressured to bottle-feed because I knew that I would be going back to work when my son was eight weeks old. He was totally breastfed until I returned to work. Then bottles of formula quickly took over. I was surprised how much that upset me."*

Feelings about Returning to Work

Returning to work may bring up a range of different feelings. If you have had some choice about the length of your maternity leave, you may feel ready to return. It may still be hard to leave your baby. Or you may feel angry, sad or guilty about having to return.

When the time came for Peggy to go back to work, she felt ready: *"Of course I missed her, but I knew she was in good hands. She still had early morning and nighttime feedings, which became very important times for me. I think that we both did well from being apart from one another. She got the stimulation and variety of other people, who had time and energy for her. I got the chance to engross myself in a great job. I came back fresh to her at the end of the day."*

Lois felt nowhere near ready to return to work after four months when she said she'd first go part time: *"I was nursing every three hours or so and Tessa wouldn't take a bottle. I wanted to keep on breastfeeding. But I saw no real way to combine it with the demands of work. I hadn't really come to terms with motherhood. I felt I had to be there all the time to be any good at it. My new manager didn't understand. She saw my indecision as lack of commitment. I resigned, feeling that a 'perfect' mother should always be there for her children. Part of me was glad to lose the pressure of work, but part wasn't. I came to resent having to stay at home. It made me more tense and Tessa felt this."*

Tamara felt that returning to work changed the focus of her relationship with her son: *"Because only I could feed and nurture him, I felt a huge sense of responsibility. It was terrible to have to leave him. Financially, we had no choice. I didn't know beforehand how I was going to feel once he was born. I felt that going back to work really damaged the closeness and intensity of our relationship. It really upset me. I also felt very guilty. That made me want to succeed with breastfeeding even more. I felt at least it was something I could do for my baby."*

Continuing to breastfeed may be a way for you to maintain the special bond you have with your baby. This is how Danielle and Barbara felt: *"When I finally went back to work, I felt breastfeeding was part of the bond I did not want to break. I nursed up until the last minute before going to work and expressed during the day."*

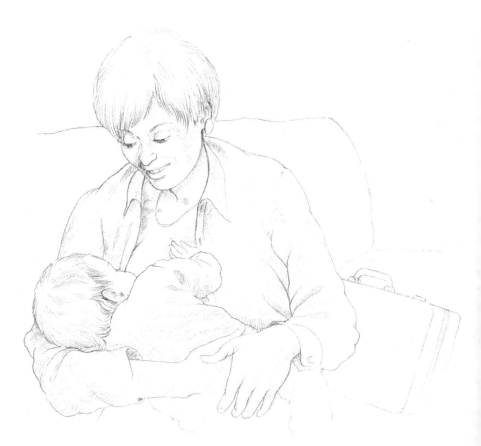

"*Besides feeling as though I was giving my daughter the best start in life, breastfeeding has given us a special closeness. For a mom who had to return to work very early on, this was extremely important to me. It has made our relationship special. I'm sharing something with her that no other caregiver can. I'm not saying that moms who don't breastfeed don't feel those special things too. Just that, for me, it was important to feel them in that way.*"

Paula was not looking forward to returning to work. She was worried how Charlotte would take to a bottle with her babysitter: *"It helped to see my little bags of breast milk filling up the freezer. I think this was my way of coming to terms with my worries about leaving Charlotte. Expressing milk was something positive I could do about a situation I could not fully control.*"

Feeding: The Options

If you are breastfeeding, you have a number of options for feeding your baby when you return to work. The choice you make depends on your own circumstances and feelings. You may decide to give your baby breast milk only. You may use both breast milk and formula milk or other drinks. Or you may decide to wean your baby from the breast. You may find it helpful to discuss these options with a breastfeeding counselor or other working mothers who have breastfed. Talking with them may help you choose what will suit you best.

If you decide to give your baby breast milk only, you may express milk to be given to your baby by her caregiver while you are away. Then you can breastfeed when you are at home. Or you may work at home, or be able to visit your baby during the day to breastfeed. Older babies may be taking other drinks and not need breast milk while you are at work. You may decide to continue breastfeeding. Or you may be prepared to stop if problems come up.

Suellen dreaded going back to work. She was breastfeeding and her daughter, Rosalyn, was thriving on it. She didn't like the idea of giving up: *"I decided I would try expressing milk to leave for her to be fed by the babysitter. After consulting my doctor, who was a great support, and various magazines and so forth, I purchased a hand pump and went to work. The results were depressing to begin with. Finally I was able to get a fair amount out (8 ounces). I also learned the best times to express.*

"I'm happy to say that I have now been back to work (part time) for four weeks. Expressing is going very well. I have a freezer full of expressed milk that has first been frozen in ice-cube trays and then transferred to freezer bags. The knowledge that I have plenty of 'backup' milk in the freezer (enough for two weeks) helps me relax when I can't express the exact amount she needs each week. Each week I arrive at the door of my babysitter with Rosalyn and a tote bag full of frozen breast milk.

"My boss is supportive in making space for me to express my milk at work twice a day. He lets me store it in the refrigerator. (No one has used it yet for their coffee, either.) Expressing does require persistence and organization. But to me it has been well worth the effort. I plan to continue for as long as is possible."

Jacqui kept on breastfeeding after returning to work part time because she enjoys nursing. Breastfeeding was well established and she didn't feel ready to break the bond: *"Both times, my kids were 10 or 11 months old before I returned to work. So I had plenty of time to build up a supply of frozen milk to leave at home. By this stage, my milk supply had settled down. Although my breasts were very full at the end of my working day, I didn't need to express milk at work. Since I only work two days a week, I kept nursing at lunchtime on my nonworking days. I had no problems in terms of milk production."*

By the time Natalie went back to work, her daughter Esther was ready for a full day at preschool: *"Esther was still nursing at noon. So for the first couple of weeks back at work, I drove over at lunch time and nursed her at the preschool. It was a bother, but I felt it got both of us used to the idea of changing our routines gradually. The preschool staff was very supportive. I never felt uncomfortable about sitting there, breastfeeding."*

You may decide to use both breast and formula milk. Perhaps you'll breastfeed at home, and use formula milk while you are working. It may be hard for you to express milk. Or you may prefer not to. Once you establish breastfeeding, you may find that your breasts, and your baby, adapt well to a combination of breast milk and formula. You may have problems with leaking or overfull breasts until your supply settles down. You may need to express a small amount of milk at work for comfort. Pressing on the nipples may help prevent leaking. This can be done discreetly if you cross your arms, but it may be a good idea to keep a spare top at work just in case.

Kelly found that both breast and bottle worked well for her: *"When I returned to work (when my first child was seven months and then when my second child was five months), I was still fully breastfeeding on my days off. It was a little uncomfortable at first, but both my body and the babies adapted quickly. I nursed them on my days off and in the morning and at night. They took a bottle of formula from their caregivers while I was working."*

Another plan is to wean your baby from the breast when you go back to work, if you are ready to finish breastfeeding or if you feel that working and breastfeeding would not be possible.

Hazel chose to stop breastfeeding when she returned to work: *"I was lucky to be able to take a long maternity break. I used maternity leave, then vacations—it really added up. By the end of this time, I was ready to stop breastfeeding."*

A job with long hours away from her baby left Naomi with no choice: *"I kept up with the evening feeding until she was 17 months old. I only stopped then because I changed jobs. Now I commute to the city. The problems of public transportation and the need to attend evening meetings mean I could not always be home to give her an evening feeding. So I decided it was better for her to have a regular bedtime routine that did not require my presence."*

If you want to breastfeed very much, you may decide to leave your job because coordinating breastfeeding and a job doesn't seem to work out.

Danielle's baby more or less led the way: *"The baby would only accept bottles of breast milk from my husband, not the babysitter! He became weak by starving himself if I wasn't there, even though he was on mixed feeding by that time. I gave up work again after a few weeks."*

Tory's boss made it clear where she stood: *"I went back to work as a cook when my baby was six weeks old. I wanted to carry on fully breastfeeding. But my boss was not helpful. I was not allowed a break to leave work and nurse the baby elsewhere. And when I expressed milk at work, I was told that the other staff were upset by what I was doing. I had to stop. My work was part time, so I had no rights. So I quit."*

Expressing Milk

You may plan to express milk, at home or at work, to meet all or most of your baby's needs. You may need to express milk at work for your own comfort, or to keep up your supply. Maintaining a supply of expressed breast milk can be a big job. If you work full time and have little or no support, the challenge is greater. Like breastfeeding, expressing milk may take practice. Often it is easier to begin to express milk before you return to work. This gives you time to experiment and decide what method of expressing works best for you. It also enables you to build up a stock of frozen milk for use later.

FEEDING FILE

Expressing milk for your baby:
Things to consider before you return to work

- Each workplace is different. You may find it useful to talk through your specific conditions with a breastfeeding counselor and your employer.

- Choosing the right pump is important. If possible, try out different types before you return to work.

- Some La Leche League newsletters carry for-sale and want ads. You may find a second-hand pump.

- See if your baby's caregiver is willing to store and carefully defrost expressed breast milk left for your baby.

- Start your baby on a bottle (or cup) before you go back to work. Someone other than you may be better. Your baby expects to breastfeed from you. She may not accept a substitute from you.

- Make a "trial run" before the first day you must leave your baby. It could turn up unforeseen problems. There may be time to change your plans.

Wendy put together her own routine at work: *"I use a breast pump at home, but at work I express by hand. It is easier for sterilizing purposes. I have my own soap and towel. I express into a sterilized milk container. Then I transfer the milk to a sterilized baby bottle that I keep in a cooler bag big enough to hold five ice packs and the bottle. I also pack the bag with bubble packaging. It is very important to have a good cooler bag and to open it only to put in the milk."*

Melanie is a full-time teacher. She found expressing easy the first time around: *"It used to take less than 30 seconds to get a let down on the pump. In the end, my babysitter and I both threw out the frozen reserves. So when it came to Greg, my second child, I didn't freeze too much in reserve. My first week back, I had a nasty shock. I was only getting 3 to 4 ounces (100 to 120ml) per pumping. Greg needed two feedings of 6 ounces (200ml) or more! I started nursing at night again, pumped three times (at lunch, 4 p.m. and 6 p.m.) and tried to rest. Five weeks later, my supply was just about keeping up with his demand."*

The most important factor when you express milk, however you do it, is to make sure your milk is letting down. This means that you are collecting the fat-rich hindmilk and not just the foremilk stored in the ducts.

BREAST PUMPS

- Breast pumps work by suction, which draws the milk out of the breast. The suction is created by hand or by electric power. The suction strength on most pumps is adjustable.

- Different pumps suit different women.

- Some pumps are easier to assemble and clean than others. You may find it useful to talk to someone with experience in pumping to learn more.

- If you buy a pump and find it doesn't work after you have given it a good try, take it back.

- Some pumps come with a soft Flexishield® plastic shield, which fits inside the rigid plastic funnel that is placed over the nipple area. The Flexishield molds around the breast. When the pump is working, the action emulates a baby sucking. This stimulates the breast so the breast-milk yield is greater.

- Flexishields are also sold separately from pumps. Contact the manufacturer, Ameda/Egnell at 1-800-323-8750, for more information.

Hand Pumps

- A simple hand pump may be enough for part-time work. They are not expensive and are easy to sterilize.

- Most hand pumps work by pressure on a lever, or by pulling a cylinder in and out.

- Lever pumps are designed for one-handed use. Some women manage to nurse their baby at one breast while they express from the other.

- All hand pumps are small and portable, and quiet to use. They are suitable for expressing at work.

- Some women complain that with frequent use, the plastic parts on hand pumps wear out.

- Don't use the type of hand pump, or "breast reliever," as it is called, that consists of a rubber bulb attached to a plastic funnel which fits over the breast. (Sometimes there is also a screw-on bottle attached.) It is hard to obtain suction by squeezing the bulb, and the pump cannot be sterilized properly.

Melanie learned this for herself: *"It appeared, even to me, that the 2 ounces (50ml) or so that I could get after half an hour without a let down must be foremilk only. The cream didn't rise to the top in the refrigerator the way it does with milk from a good pumping session.*

"The books suggest that you look at a picture of the baby, fix your mind on his little head and think milk. What has to happen for me is to get so engrossed in the paper, or a crossword puzzle, or in talking to my husband after work, that I don't think about it. Then the milk lets down."

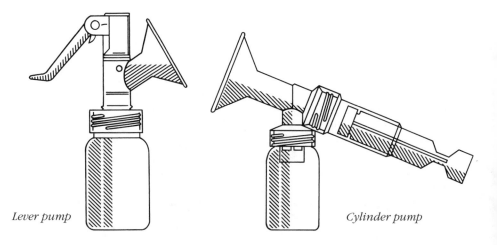

Lever pump   *Cylinder pump*

Rita sometimes had to encourage her let down: *"If I'm very engorged, I have no problems expressing milk. But if I have trouble starting, I nurse the baby on the other side. It can be awkward, trying to support him and express at the same time. But often it works. Standing under a shower also can start a let down."*

Facilities and support for breastfeeding mothers at the workplace vary. It helps to contact your employer in advance to make sure there is someplace you can express milk at work.

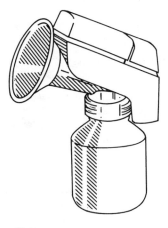

Battery pump

Jinny was lucky with her employer: *"I decided for many reasons that I wanted to keep nursing after I went back to work. I felt it was still some part of me that I could give to him even though I couldn't be there with him all day. And now he was being exposed to more germs and other children. I felt that the antibodies in my milk were helping his immune system develop. It was also my way of reminding myself and others that even if I was back at work, being a mother came first.*

BREAST PUMPS

Electric pumps

- Electric pumps are powered by battery or 110V. Some use either.

- Pumps range from small, lightweight, hand-held battery pumps to larger electric models weighing from 5 to 20 lbs. that rest on a table.

- Prices vary. Small battery pumps are cheapest. Large electric pumps can cost from $75 to $110, plus running costs. Large hospital-quality pumps cost more. They can often be rented.

- Suction strength varies with the size of the pump. A small battery pump may not help you to express more milk than a hand pump, but it may be less tiring.

- Batteries run down quickly with regular use. Rechargeable batteries and a charger are good investments.

- Large electric pumps have attachments for expressing both breasts at once. Dual pumping is faster and can increase the amount you get.

- Electric pumps make some noise.

- The Egnell 'Elite' is a new electric pump that is light and easy to use.

- Large electric pumps may be rented locally from "Pump Stations." For the Pump Station nearest you, call Medela at 1-800-435-8316 or Ameda/Egnell at 1-800-323-8750. Or call La Leche League, at 1-800-LA LECHE or 1-847-519-9585, weekdays between 8 a.m. and 5 p.m., Central Time.

- Your insurance company may cover the rental cost of a good-quality pump. A prescription for breastmilk must be written by a doctor *in the baby's name.* A prescription for a breast pump written in the mother's name is not likely to be covered.

"I had a great time. Although I worked in a very male-oriented profession, as a petroleum engineer in an oil field, I found my co-workers and bosses very supportive. I had a great electric dual breast pump. I would take 15-minute morning and afternoon breaks. I could easily pump 18-22 ounces. I had a private office, but no lock. And we had a refrigerator/freezer in the coffee bar. There were quite a few good-natured jokes from my co-workers, especially about my full breasts right before 'milking,' as they called it. But I didn't feel offended. They seemed to adopt my son as the department mascot. I found it so relaxing to take those 15-minute breaks, to think about Josh and to let go of any stress at work. I knew that what I was doing was very important."

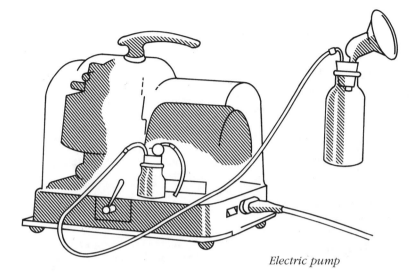

Electric pump

Carla had a slightly different, but also supportive experience: *"I told my immediate supervisor that I wanted to have somewhere to go and express my milk. He arranged for me to go to the nurse's room. I express twice a day. I don't use the refrigerator at work. It might bother the other workers to open the refrigerator and find human milk. Also, if you keep your milk by your side all day, you are sure not to forget it. I keep mine in a cooler underneath my desk."*

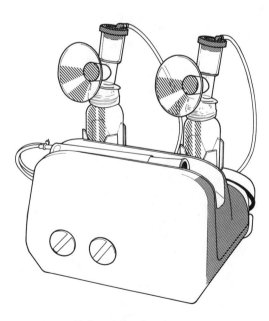

Lightweight electric pump

FEEDING FILE

Expressing Milk by Hand

The good

- No special equipment is needed, only a wide-necked sterile container and clean hands.

- Hand expressing is closer to a baby's sucking than expressing by pump. It may be a better way to maintain your milk supply.

- Expressing by hand may be gentler than expressing with a pump.

The bad

- It may take longer to express by hand than by pump.

- Your hands may get tired.

How to hand express

- Use a hand to cup your breast from underneath. Put your forefinger along the line where your areola (the dark part around your nipple) and breast meet. Place your thumb on top of your breast, along the same line.

- Your milk is stored in reservoirs a bit below this line. These reservoirs need to be squeezed gently to extract the milk. You may need to move your hand slightly in towards your nipple or back towards your chest to find the milk reservoirs. Experiment until you find the right place for you.

- Gently squeeze your thumb and fingers together, pushing back and in towards your ribcage at the same time. These movements help push the milk along the ducts towards the nipple, as well as squeezing it out.

- Relax the pressure, then repeat the movements.

- Your milk may take a minute or two to begin flowing. Don't give up if nothing happens right away.

- Move your hand around your breast, so that you cover all the milk ducts. You could also change hands on the same breast.

- If your hand gets tired, change sides. Come back to the first side later.

- Sometimes it is easier to learn to hand express after you have been shown how. A lactation counselor or La Leche League leader should be able to help you.

- The very best way to learn may be to watch someone who can do it. Ask a lactation counselor or a La Leche League leader if she knows some-one who might show you how.

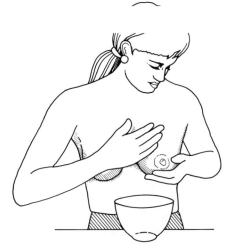

Stroking the entire breast, working from the ribcage towards the nipple area, will help the milk flow.

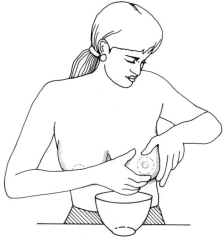

Cup your breast from underneath, with your forefinger along the line where your areola and breast meet. Place your thumb on top of the same line.

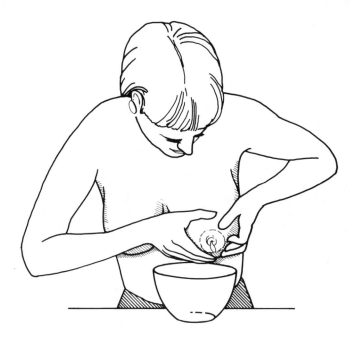

Gently squeeze your thumb and fingers together, pushing back and in towards your ribcage.

FEEDING FILE

Tips for Expressing Milk

- Expressing gets easier and more productive with practice. Don't worry if you get only a little milk at first.

- The best time to express varies from person to person. There may be a time when your breasts feel fuller, perhaps early morning. Once you return to work, a routine of expressing may be imposed by coffee-breaks and work schedule.

- When you are learning, try to choose a time when you are not rushed and won't be interrupted.

- A warm, comfortable place with a comfortable chair works best.

- Being relaxed helps the milk to flow, so think about what helps you relax. You might listen to music or do relaxation exercises first.

- Stroke the whole breast. Work from the rib cage towards the nipple area. This helps get the milk to flow.

- Think about your baby and your milk flowing. Sometimes it helps to have a photo of your baby nearby or to play an audiotape of him.

- Back massage may help the milk flow. If there is someone who can do this, get him or her to stand behind you, with a fist either side of your spine, level with your breasts. Rub the fists up and down, gently but firmly.

- Warmth can help the milk flow. Try expressing after a bath or shower. Or try putting a warm wash cloth on your breast. Or hug a hot-water bottle.

- Some mothers find it is helpful to think of other things to get their milk flowing. A TV show, a book or some good conversation may help.

- Try expressing from one breast while your baby nurses from the other. Or keep expressing just after nursing.

How much milk to express

- It can be hard to know how much expressed milk your baby will need while you are away.

- Allow 2-$\frac{1}{2}$ ounces of milk for each pound of the baby's weight in 24 hours. For example, a 10-pound baby might take 25 ounces of milk in 24 hours. This is a very rough guide. Breastfed babies may take more or less than this. And their intake may not be even throughout the day.

- When you have been back at work for a week or two, you will have a better idea of how much milk your baby needs. Even so, extra milk in the refrigerator or freezer is a useful "backup" in case your baby's needs increase suddenly.

FEEDING FILE

Storing Expressed Breast Milk

- Use fresh, rather than frozen, breast milk whenever you can. Freezing has some effect on the nutrients and immune properties of breast milk.

- Expressed milk can be stored in a refrigerator for 24 hours or in a deep freeze for up to 3 months. You may read elsewhere that longer storage times are OK. We are being cautious here.

- Store milk in the coldest part of the refrigerator, often the back or bottom. It may be worth buying a fridge thermometer. Breast milk should be stored at 39°F or below.

- After expressing, cool milk quickly in a container of cold water. Then store it in the refrigerator. An insulated cooler with ice packs can work if you do not have access to a fridge at work. You can use the same cooler to transport fresh or frozen milk to your baby's caregiver.

- To freeze milk, cool it quickly first. Then freeze it in sterile plastic bags or lidded plastic containers, labeled and dated. Covered plastic ice-cube trays can be used for freezing. Then move the cubes to another container for storage.

- Don't fill containers too full. Leave room for expansion during freezing.

- Freeze your milk in small amounts. Then you won't have to defrost, and perhaps waste, more milk than your baby needs.

- Freshly expressed milk can be added to milk expressed or frozen earlier. But cool the new milk separately first. And don't add more than half the amount of milk already frozen to a pre-frozen batch.

- Defrost frozen breast milk as quickly as you can. Hold the container under cool, then warmer, running water. Or stand it in hot water. Use the same method for warming expressed milk or use a bottle warmer.

- Don't use a microwave to thaw or warm milk. The milk may overheat, or heat unevenly, and some nutrients will be destroyed.

- Thawed milk that has *not* been heated may be stored in the refrigerator for 24 hours. But throw out any unused milk that was warmed.

- If the fat separates during storage, shake the milk container.

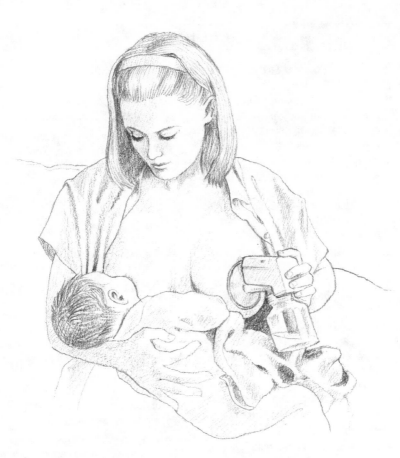

Starting with Cups or Bottles

Many babies adapt well to taking expressed breast milk, formula or other drinks by bottle or cup from their caregiver. They breastfeed when you are there. A cup may be better than a bottle for babies who may become confused by the different sucking actions needed for breast and bottle. Some breastfed babies are reluctant to take a bottle. You may have to be persistent. It can help to try different nipples, or to warm the nipple. Someone other than you may be better at getting your baby to take a bottle. Your baby connects you with breastfeeding.

About six weeks before going back to work, when her baby was about six months old, Natalie started to cut down on the number of breast-feedings. She wanted her baby to get used to having fewer breastfeedings throughout the day: *"I tried replacing breastfeedings with fruit juice and water, water, formula milk, cow's milk or expressed breast milk. I tried cups with various types of spouts and bottles with various types of nipples. Nothing worked. She never took a bottle. And at this stage her cup skills were pretty basic. When we got down to three feedings a day, I was reluctant to drop further feedings. I didn't feel she was drinking enough. The staff at the day care told me she only took mouthfuls of fluids compared to the 8-ounce bottles of milk the others were having. I was worried that she'd get dehydrated or constipated. Or that she'd start to wake up in the night wanting more feedings. I knew that she must be getting enough fluids. But I worried because she hardly seemed to be drinking anything."*

Paula's daughter, Charlotte, would only accept breast milk from the breast: *"Once I was back at work, I found that Charlotte wasn't going to take breast milk from a bottle or a cup or a spoon. Instead, I used breast milk to mix up baby rice. Then I stirred the rice mixture into fruit and vegetable purées."*

Rita's baby was happy to take her milk from a bottle: *"I began to express milk early on. Once or twice each week my husband slept downstairs with the baby and gave him a bottle of my milk. It meant that I was able to get six or seven hours of unbroken sleep. The baby had a bottle often enough to get used to it, but not too often to break the routine of nursing from me."*

The Need for Support

In an ideal world, all working mothers would have a longer period of paid maternity leave. When they went back to work, they'd have the option of flexible working hours or part-time work. Breastfeeding mothers would have the right to breastfeeding or expressing breaks during the work day. There would be more childcare at the workplace or nearby. And there would be nice, private places to express milk at work. Some mothers do manage to put together decent arrangements for themselves and enjoy the support of family, friends and employers.

Wendy's husband was her greatest support: *"On the whole, it has worked out fine, even better than if my husband had gone to work and I had stayed at home. It is less tiring to go to work than to look after a baby and do the housework. What has made the whole thing so easy is the fact that my husband has been very supportive. He really did everything at home. Also, we slept with the baby in our bed, which is good for the baby, good for me because I need to be with her, and good for my sleep, too. Despite working full time, I am with my baby 16 hours a day."*

Tessa returned to work as a full-time nurse working shifts when her baby was five months old: *"The baby nursed at 5:30 a.m. I left for work at 6 a.m., having packed a supply of breast milk for Owen while he's at day care. My husband was a full-time student in his last year. He took Owen to day care in the morning and I picked him up at 4:30 p.m. when I finished work. When I worked on a late shift until 9:30 p.m., I took Owen to day care and my husband picked him up after his classes. When I got him at 4:30 p.m., I breastfed him again before taking him home. We live in a town 30 miles from the day care, not a five-minute trip, and he couldn't wait. At home I nursed him on demand the rest of the evening and night. Because he nursed on one side, I pumped and stored (refrigerated or froze) the milk from the other side.*

"The baby was up every two hours to nurse at night and wanted to suck all evening when we got home. This was on top of a day at work and shopping, housework, and all that. My husband wasn't really able to help with shopping and housework because he was taking his final exams. I had to really work to make it succeed! Every time the baby nursed at night, it was not a case of a quick feeding and back to sleep. I had to force myself to get up, pump the milk from the other side, store it or freeze it, and resterilize all the pumping things for the next time. After that, I climbed back into bed.

"I had really wanted to breastfeed to give my baby the best start in life. And I was determined to keep nursing when I went back to work. He nursed well. Thankfully, that was not a problem. I loved breastfeeding. Although it was tough at the time, I consider it a great achievement on my part that my baby continued with breast milk while I worked full time."

Combining breastfeeding and work can be demanding. The challenge is greatest for mothers who work full time and whose babies are fully breastfed. Good support from others who have done or are doing the same helps. Helpful employers, people who will help with chores, and above all, people who think that it is worth all the effort, can also make things much easier.

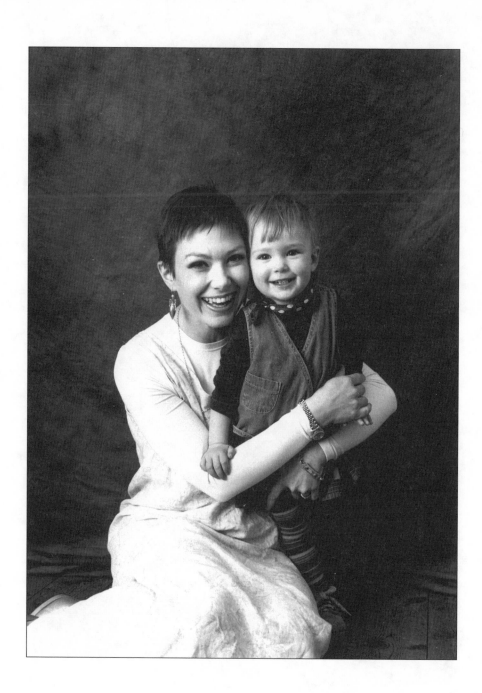

CHAPTER 12 *Finishing Breastfeeding*

Finishing breastfeeding ends a very special relationship between a mother and her baby. You may finish almost as soon as you have started because of too many problems. Or you may just decide it is not for you. You may have breastfed for many months but reached the stage where your baby or you are ready to stop. However long you breastfeed, there is no doubt that it will have created a unique bond. Breastfeeding may also have brought other rewards, such as a sense of fulfillment and achievement, and a boost to self-confidence. You may have mixed feelings when you stop breastfeeding and a new stage in your baby's life begins, as these three mothers did:

"My time as a breastfeeding mother is something I'll always remember with great pleasure. I was lucky to have few problems. But I found weaning hard. The books say you drop one feeding one week, substitute other food or drinks, then another, until the baby is weaned. But my daughter didn't want anything except breastmilk. We finally did it, but it was a struggle."

"Part of me misses the special closeness of breastfeeding and the ability to comfort her instantly."

"Two days after the last feeding, I just could not stop crying. A friend told me that 'weaning grief' was common and didn't mean I was wrong to stop breastfeeding. I wish I had known about this before. I did not understand it and was afraid it was the start of delayed postpartum depression. But the next day I felt normal again."

Regrets may be stronger if your baby chooses to stop nursing before you had planned. Cindy enjoyed nursing Beth. She remembers vividly the first feeding she refused at five or six months: *"It was at lunchtime. I felt rejected and sad that my little baby was becoming independent."*

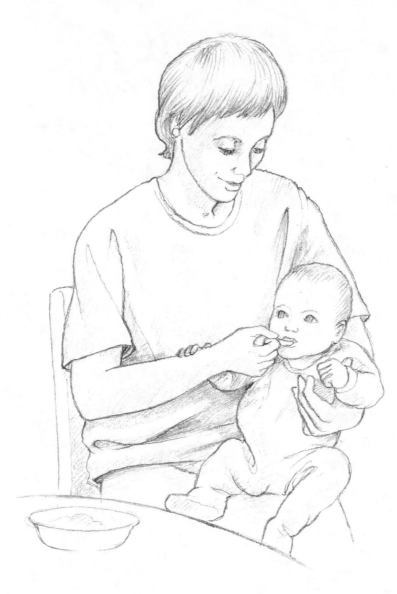

Joanna's first baby suddenly refused to nurse when he was about nine months old: *"It was very hard on me. I had only heard and read about deciding when you wanted to stop nursing or trying to stop when the baby wanted to continue. It was also a physical problem for me. He was a baby who had been very reluctant to eat solid food. He was still taking four or five large feedings a day from me."*

You may be happy to stop breastfeeding. You may have nursed for as long as you wanted and are ready to move on.

Jane's baby is now nine months: *"Over the last three weeks or so, I've cut down on breastfeeding so that she often just has a feeding at bed-time—7 p.m. I'm happy with this. I'm looking forward to stopping—a feeling I'm surprised at. I thought I'd be reluctant to stop nursing our last baby."*

Sometimes it may be a relief to stop breastfeeding, especially if the experience has not been a good one.

Kate was advised by her doctor to stop breastfeeding and change to formula feedings: *"Well, it would be wrong to say that everything was rosy from that day onward. But I can honestly say that things did improve. I no longer had this baby sucking at me all the time. And I got to sleep for a few hours at a time rather than minutes. I am positive that if I had kept up the breastfeeding struggle it would have taken a lot longer for my daughter and me to develop the fantastic relationship we now have, if at all."*

Who Chooses When to Stop?

The best time to start weaning your baby from the breast depends on your feelings and your own breastfeeding circumstances. Sometimes your baby leads the way with weaning. She begins to lose interest in breastfeeding as she grows older and is distracted by other things.

Jill found weaning a fairly natural process. *"After five months, I found that his attention was moving to the outside world. He constantly moved off the breast at the slightest distraction. So I nursed him at quiet times (morning, evening and during the night if necessary). But I gave him a bottle during the day when there were more distractions. By seven months, he began to lose interest and dropped the evening feeding. And finally at eight months, he no longer wanted the breast at all. I was very pleased that he had chosen when to stop nursing. But I know that he may have done this more quickly because he was also getting a bottle."*

Anna's daughter waited a bit longer before making her feelings clear: *"When she was 14 months old, she sat on my lap one bedtime and said 'juice.' I obeyed her clear command. She settled down. The following evening I offered my slightly over-full breast and she had a last feeding. We both seemed to know it was a savored closeness."*

You may decide yourself when to begin weaning your baby from the breast. You may have nursed for as long as you want to, or you may have other reasons. You may be returning to work or wanting to get pregnant. You may even be influenced by comments from friends or relatives.

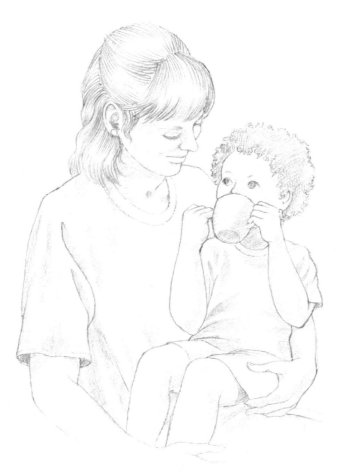

These influences can be positive, as they were for Jean: *"I thought about weaning Roberta at four months. One new friend was breastfeeding her second child. The fact that she was still happily nursing her baby at six months gave me courage to withstand comments such as 'You're still nursing?'"*

Anne-Marie's family was less positive: *"My mother and sister thought I was a fanatic about breastfeeding. They kept asking why was I putting myself and my baby through all this. My mom nursed me for six weeks and then she didn't have enough milk. So she couldn't understand why I was so against formula. My sister had used supplemental bottles and had finally switched to bottle-feeding with her two children. The pressure was subtle. I doubt they knew how upsetting it was. But I got their 'message' loud and clear."*

It helps to share how you feel about stopping breastfeeding with your partner. Kirsty and her husband saw breastfeeding in different ways: *"Together, my husband, Sandy, and I decided that I'd stop breastfeeding during our summer vacation. Jim would be 17 months old. Sandy saw Jim's breastfeeding as a habit to be broken. I saw it as a part of our relationship. It was intimate and fulfilling for both of us. When I stopped nursing, both my mind and body ached to nurse Jim again. But with each feeding refused, Sandy felt that I was one step nearer my goal. Having a different idea of breastfeeding from my husband and not talking about this openly and early enough was one of the things that made stopping much harder than it needed to be."*

Angela's daughter, Carol, was weaned from the breast on the advice of her doctor: *"I didn't want to stop breastfeeding, but I was deeply depressed. My doctor advised me to wean her for my health's sake. I reluctantly agreed that it might help. I don't remember it upsetting her as much as I had expected. But I decided to give her a bottle in the evenings. She'd always been a 'sucky' baby, but had never sucked her thumb. It was hard to suddenly deprive her of her comfort habit."*

Some babies don't mind replacing breastfeedings with other drinks or food, or do not object to being diverted from nursing.

Ruth started to wean Lily slowly at about five months. She took solids very well. As she had more solids, she began to reduce breastfeedings: *"I cut out the morning feeding first. I decreased the sucking time one minute at a time. Once the morning feeding was gone, I went on to cut out the night feeding. Although it was my decision to stop nursing completely, I did miss the closeness and warmth of breastfeeding my baby. For a few weeks, it was as though Lily didn't need me any more. She didn't bat an eyelid at not being breastfed. I am grateful, though, that it was a gradual process and not traumatic at all."*

Some babies are reluctant to be weaned from the breast. Sometimes older babies and toddlers become determined breastfeeders. You and your partner may need to devise strategies to help your child accept the end of breastfeeding. Substitutes will be needed for the comfort and security your baby or child has gained from breastfeeding, as well as for the breast milk itself.

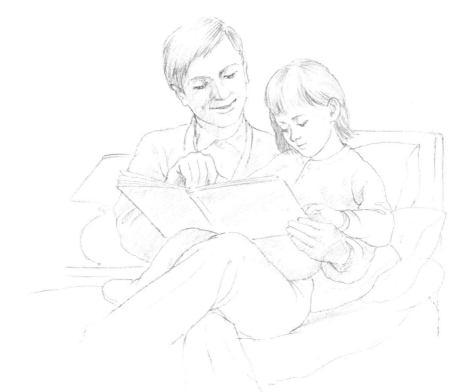

Christine and her husband worked together to get their son to change his pattern: *"When I finally decided it was time to start weaning my son from the breast, he had other ideas. He was eating and drinking plenty of other things. But breastfeeding was still important to him—in the morning, at nap time and at bedtime. My husband put him to bed for a week while I made myself scarce. That ended the bedtime feeding. At nap time, I took to pushing him in the stroller, rather than sitting down on the sofa with him as I had done before. The morning feeding was hardest. It took place at about 5:30 a.m. and gave us all some extra rest. I didn't want to make myself scarce by getting up so early. So this feeding continued until I got pregnant again. Then we started putting Chris to bed later. He began to wake later in the morning. At that point I could face getting up and making breakfast, rather than nursing."*

Bedtime was the toughest time for Polly: *"As John grew older, he began to drink juice during the day. But I couldn't work out how to put a baby to bed without nursing. He still fell asleep at the breast. I needed the morning feeding to remove the milk I produced during the night. By the time he was 16 months old, we were down to two feedings a day for months. But we were no closer to dropping them. Nick had always bathed John. We dried and dressed him between us, then I nursed him before going to bed. We finally agreed that for the next week, I would hide during the bath. Nick would put him to bed. This worked in just a week. It took longer for the milk supply to dry up, and I lived on painkillers for about three days. So much for the people who said John couldn't be taking much milk at his age, and was just comfort-sucking!"*

Stopping Because of Problems

Many women stop breastfeeding not because they feel ready to wean the baby, but because they are having problems that do not seem easy to resolve. For some women, the pain (both physical and emotional) connected with breastfeeding is just too much to bear. They decide, often with mixed feelings, to add formula feedings to breastfeeding. Starting formula because of problems may lead to the end of breast-feeding completely, as these mothers discovered:

"By the end of the second week, the cracked nipple had not healed. I was bleeding when nursing or using the breast pump. I would have stuck with it, but my baby was fussy and seemed very hungry. That's when I decided to give him a bottle. He turned into a different baby, very happy and much more content. I was really disappointed at what I saw as my failure to breastfeed. But I felt that he would be a happier baby if I finished his feeding with a bottle. I slowly increased bottles and decreased breast. I stopped breastfeeding completely when my son was six weeks old."

"After a really grim evening when the baby had been trying to nurse for about five hours, my husband made the decision for me that we had to bottle-feed. I couldn't have decided for myself. I would have felt too guilty. By then the baby was 10 days old. He had not had one good breastfeeding. He drank the formula like crazy, and hasn't looked back since. I expressed milk as much as I could. But after only three weeks it dried up, which really disappointed me."

If you have stopped nursing because of problems, you may be left with very strong feelings—of disappointment, failure, guilt, anger or sadness.

Stopping breastfeeding was an emotional time for Celia: *"After 4-½ weeks, I finally gave in and went to bottle-feeding. I felt totally depressed and a complete failure as a mom. I was sad that no one seemed to have any advice that could have helped me over those first tough weeks. My sense of failure was great. The guilt that I had given in where others seemed to have persevered is still with me now. I was very envious of all breastfeeding moms. I also feel that if I had had access to greater support in the form of other moms who were breastfeeding or had breastfed, I would have been able to continue."*

Stopping breastfeeding made sense to Debbie. But emotionally she was less sure: *"Bottles allowed me independence. They gave me stretches of time when I could feed myself and think about other things. To that point I had rarely left the baby except to go to the bathroom. Life was easier, except for preparing formula milk. But my guilt and feelings of failure are still with me. I did not feel any sense of love for my baby when she was born. I was very anxious that nothing should be wrong with her. Afterwards I felt sick with responsibility. Through breastfeeding, I was able to bond with my daughter and grow to love her. Now, when I can't feed her myself and see her hands on the bottle I am upset because I wish they were holding on to me."*

Connie's decision was caused by illness, but it was no less hard for her: *"At four months, I got a stomach virus. I was admitted to the hospital with dehydration. I decided to stop nursing because I was exhausted. I expressed milk for a few days until I made my decision. This also eased the pain and leakage from my engorged breasts. It was a very sad time for me. Not only did I miss my baby, I felt I had failed. We live at the other end of the country from our families. So there was no one to help or put things in perspective then."*

It seems as though these women felt their lack of success with breastfeeding was a failure. These are common feelings. You may accept them and go on to hope you might be able to "get it right" next time. You may feel guilty. If you choose to breastfeed and are not able to, then yes, there has been a failure. But does it mean *you* have failed? Surely not.

You need help and support to succeed at breastfeeding. If help and support is not available or is not skilled, and you do not succeed with breastfeeding, could the fault lie with the system of support? These mothers think so.

Shelly's main feeling is one of anger that the help she had was so poor: *"Having talked to other mothers, I know now that my problem wasn't uncommon. With the right advice it could have been resolved. Everyone placed so much emphasis on breastfeeding before birth. But when the time, came no one seemed to have the skills needed to make it work. I began to wonder if they'd received any training in breastfeeding."*

Sandra feels bitter that she didn't have the support she needed when trying to breastfeed her first two children: *"It seems to me too many of the health providers that I met were too ready to advise the bottle at the first sign of any problems. They didn't give realistic support to help me succeed at nursing. In other words, all the advice that seemed to be there is built around giving up a sorry attempt. I heard things like . . . 'formula is so good these days that when she is a year old, you won't be able to tell whether she was breast- or bottle-fed.' I allowed myself to believe this the first time. But now that I know I can breastfeed successfully, I feel cheated."*

Amanda assumed her new baby would be bottle-fed. She had not been able to breastfeed her first baby, Jo, but: *"As time went on, I began to find out more about how to make breastfeeding work. To my horror, I learned that my inability to nurse Jo was due to what happened in the hospital. My biggest mistake was assuming that the hospital staff knew and cared enough about breastfeeding to give me the information and support I needed."*

An unhappy breastfeeding experience can be a major source of distress. You may find it helpful to contact a lactation counselor to talk over what happened. But remember, however long or short your breastfeeding experience, you gave your child the best start in life.

FEEDING FILE

Weaning Your Baby from the Breast

When to wean

- There is no right age or stage at which to begin weaning or to stop breastfeeding completely. The decision depends on the feelings and circumstances of each breast-feeding pair.

- If possible, don't start at times that may be stressful for you or your baby. Two examples might be when you return to work or when she is teething.

- It may help to discuss your plans for weaning, and your feelings about it, with a doctor or lactation counselor.

What should substitute for breast milk?

- This will depend on the age and preferences of your baby. Milk is an important source of nutrition throughout your baby's first two years.

- If you stop breastfeeding before your baby is a year old, he will probably need some formula milk. ***Cow's milk is not recommended*** for drinks until babies are a year old. But whole cow's milk can be used in cooking and with cereal.

- If your baby is eating solids and still nursing a bit, you could satisfy his thirst at other times with cooled, boiled water or well-diluted fruit juice.

- Many experts feel that "older baby formulas," advertised for babies 6 months and older, have no real advantage over other types of formula. They are also more expensive.[62]

Starting to wean

- If there is a time of day when your baby seems to care less about breastfeeding, start by cutting down or dropping that feeding. Perhaps begin at lunch time, when he has something else to eat.

- Don't start with a feeding that is an important source of comfort for your baby, such as his bedtime feeding.

- If your baby doesn't want to take formula milk in a bottle from you, someone else may have more success. She connects you with breastfeeding. You can also try different nipples. Or soften the bottle nipple in boiled water.

- Unless you need to wean your baby quickly, wait a few days or weeks between each feeding you drop. This will give both of you time to adjust.

How to replace the emotional benefits of breastfeeding

- You may need to help your baby find other ways to obtain the comfort, security and closeness he gets from breastfeeding. Some things that may help are:

  – a soft toy, special piece of clothing or blanket he can cuddle;

  – extra cuddling and stroking from you and others whom he loves;

  – at bedtime, a lullaby or a story instead of nursing.

FEEDING FILE (continued)

Bottles or cups?

- The choice of a bottle, a training cup with a spout or a normal cup for your baby depends on his age and preference.

- If he is being weaned from the breast completely, or if he is only a few months old, he may want the comfort of sucking from a bottle.

- If she is older and will be partially breastfeeding for a while, your baby may be happy to take her other drinks from a normal cup or a training cup with a lid.

- Some babies become good at drinking from a small training cup or a normal cup from about 3 or 4 months. This may be helpful if they refuse a bottle.

Babies who don't want to stop breastfeeding

- Some babies choose to stop nursing themselves. But others are extremely reluctant to stop, particularly older babies and toddlers who nurse often.

- You may need to devise strategies to help your baby stop nursing in the least stressful way.

- If possible, try to start at a time when there will be extra help or diversions. Summer may be a good time, when your child can play outside. Or try when your partner or other supportive person can be around.

- Think about the times when your child most often wants to nurse. Change your routine, so that familiar prompts and situations for breastfeeding are gone. For example, if you normally sit together on the sofa for a feeding before his nap, go out with the stroller instead.

- If it is hard to cut out feedings, start by making them shorter.

- In the morning, get up for an early breakfast instead of nursing, if you or your partner can stand it.

- At night, your partner or someone else who is close to your child could put him to bed while you go out.

- The hardest time may be during the night, when there are no other distractions and everyone needs to sleep. Your partner or another adult whom your child knows well could go to your child and comfort him for as long as necessary.

- Some mothers go away for the night or weekend when ending night feedings. Leaving your child to cry, but going regularly to reassure him, is a stressful strategy for all concerned. But it might work if all else fails.

FEEDING FILE (continued)

Weaning and you

- If possible, gradual weaning is better. Cut out a feeding every few days or weeks, or less often. This will give your body time to adjust to producing less milk. And it will cut down on the chance of over-full, sore breasts.

- Gradual weaning allows a slower decline in the level of the hormone prolactin that is produced during breastfeeding. A sudden drop in prolactin levels can sometimes lead to feelings of depression.

- If your breasts become full and hard at any time during weaning, because you are producing more milk than your baby needs now, it may help to:

  - Take a hot bath or shower, or use warm wash cloths on your breasts to encourage a small amount of milk to leak from the breasts.

  - Express just enough milk to relieve the fullness until you start to produce less milk.

  - Very gently massage your breasts towards the nipples to keep them free of lumps.

  - Use cold compresses or cabbage leaves inside your bra to relieve soreness and reduce swelling.

  - Take painkillers (but not aspirin).

  - Use any of the suggestions in chapter 4 for relieving breast fullness.

Where to get help with weaning

People to talk to:

- Your pediatric or family nurse-practitioner

- Your pediatrician or family physician

- A lactation consultant

- A La Leche League leader

- Other mothers who have breastfed and weaned their babies.

Suggested reading:

The Womanly Art of Breastfeeding. La Leche League International, 1991.

The Future

Breastfeeding mothers need better service. Public and private efforts are at work to improve the care and support of breastfeeding mothers and to improve public knowledge about the value of breastfeeding. These include training for healthcare providers, preparing or updating local breastfeeding policies, raising public awareness of breastfeeding, research, and preparing good information on breastfeeding for mothers. The future looks brighter for breastfeeding. These three mothers have the last word:

"I enjoyed nursing my two daughters very much. And I want to tell other mothers about these feelings of satisfaction and pleasure. To me, there is no greater bond between mother and child, nothing more pleasurable than nursing your own baby. It's great to be able to comfort her with the breast right away and see your baby grow bigger every week, knowing it's all your own work!"

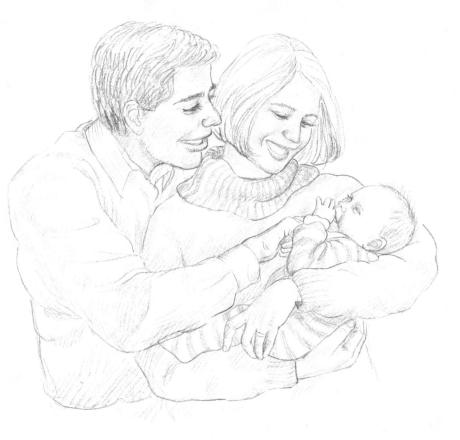

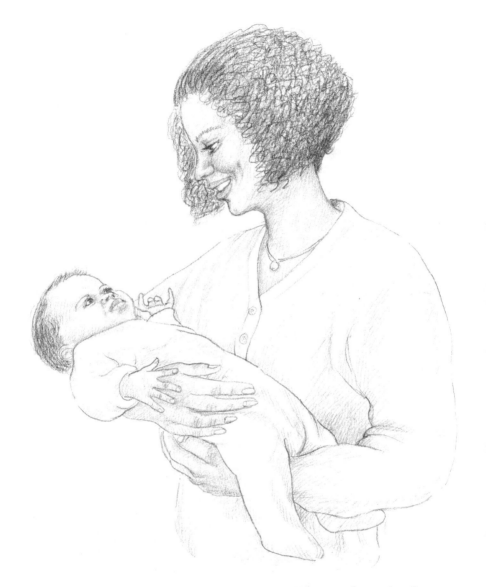

"Breastfeeding my children from almost helpless, unfocused infants, into demonstrative little people who show their obvious enjoyment and preference for the gorgeous, sweet milk was a fantastic experience."

"My breastfeeding experience has been one of the most rewarding things in my life. To know that I gave my three children the best start they could have and to have enjoyed it so much myself is at the top of my feelings about motherhood."

Where to Get Help

Breastfeeding Help and Counseling

La Leche League International
1400 North Meacham Road
Schaumburg, IL 60173-4840
(847) 519-7730

La Leche League Canada
18C Industrial Drive
P.O. Box 29
Chesterville, Ont. K0C 1H0
(613) 448-1842

La Leche League Canada Français
Secretariat General de la LLL
C.P. 874 Ville St. Laurent
Quebec, H4L 4W3
(514) 747-9127

La Leche League is a nonprofit organization. It will refer you to trained leaders and support groups nearest you. La Leche League groups hold a series of meetings for pregnant and nursing mothers. The League's Center for Breastfeeding Information can provide up-to-date information on most breastfeeding issues. The League publishes a number of helpful pamphlets on common topics. They can also help you find a breast pump that works well for you.

International Lactation Consultant Association (ILCA)
200 North Michigan Ave.
Suite 300
Chicago, IL 60601-3821
(312) 541-1710

The ILCA will refer you to a certified lactation consultant in your area.

The UNICEF Baby-friendly Hospital Initiative (BFHI):

Wellstart International
Corporate Headquarters
4062 First Ave.
San Diego, CA 92103
(619) 295-5192 (telephone)
(619) 294-7787 (fax)
or,

Wellstart International
U.S. Committee for UNICEF
Baby-friendly Hospital Initiative
4443 Pecan Valley Rd.
Nashville, TN 37218

Baby-friendly Hospital Initiative
UNICEF Canada
433 Mt. Pleasant Rd.
Toronto, Ont. M4S 2L8
(416) 482-4444 (telephone)
(416) 482-8035 (fax)

UNICEF stands for United Nations Infant and Children's Education Fund.

Support for Parents

Twin Services
P.O. Box 10066
Berkeley, CA 94709
(510) 524-0863 (telephone)
(510) 524-0894 (fax)

Twin Services offers counseling, information and referral services for the care of twins or triplets.

Provincial/Territorial Ministries of Health, Canada

Alberta
Barbara Hansen, Manager
Health Sector Development Unit
Health Planning Branch
Alberta Health
24th floor
10025 Jasper Ave.
Edmonton, AB T5J 2P
(403) 427-2653 (telephone)
(403) 427-2511 (fax)

British Columbia
Molly Butler
Prevention and Health Promotion
  Branch
Ministry of Health
Main floor
1520 Bianshard St.
Victoria, B.C. V8W 3C8
(604) 952-1531 (telephone)
(604) 952-1570 (fax)

Manitoba
Lynn Baker
Perinatal Consultant
Program Development Branch
Manitoba Health
599 Empress St.
Room 259, Second floor
Box 925
Winnipeg, Manitoba R3C 2T6
(204) 786-7305 (telephone)
(204) 772-2943 (fax)

New Brunswick
June Kerry
Department of Health and
    Community Services
P.O. Box 5100
Fredericton, NB E3B 5G8
(506) 453-2933 (telephone)
(506) 453-2726 (fax)

Newfoundland
Lynn Vivian-Book
Provincial Consultant
Parent and Child Health
Community Health
Department of Health
Confederation Building, West Block
P.O. Box 8700
St. John's, NF A1B 4J4
(709) 729-3110 (telephone)
(709) 729-5824 (fax)

Northwest Territories
Elsie De Roose
Infant/Child Nutrition Consultant
Child/Family Support Division
Department of Health and
    Social Services
Government of the Northwest
    Territories
5th floor, Precambrian Bldg. 6
P.O. Box 1320
Yellowknife, NWT X1A 2L9
(403) 873-7054 (telephone)
(403) 873-7706 (fax)

Nova Scotia
Elizabeth Shears
Public Health Services
Health Promotion Division
Nova Scotia Department of Health
1690 Hollis St., 11th floor
P.O. Box 488
Halifax, NS B3J 2R8
(902) 424-5011 (telephone)
(902) 424-0558 (fax)

Ontario
Erica Di Ruggiero
Health Promotion Branch
Population Health and Community
Services Systems Group
Ministry of Health
5700 Yonge Street, 5th floor
Toronto, Ont. M2M 4K5
(416) 314-5485 (telephone)
(416) 314-5497 (fax)

Prince Edward Island
Debra Keays
Nursing Services Coordinator
Health and Community
    Services Agency
4 Sydney St.
P.O. Box 2000
Charlottestown, PEI C1A 7N8
(902) 368-6522 (telephone)
(902) 368-6136 (fax)

Quebec
Lucille Rocheleau
Fédération des Centres locales
    de santé communautaire
1801, de Maisonneuve ouest
Pièce 600
Montréal, Quebec H3H 1J9
(514) 931-1448 (telephone)
(514) 931-9577 (fax)

Saskatchewan
Mary Scott/Myrna Dirk
Maternal and Child Health Consultant
Population Health Branch
Saskatchewan Health
3475 Albert St.
Regina, SK S4S 6X6
(306) 787-7113/787-7110 (telephone)
(306) 787-7095 (fax)

Yukon
Marnie Willis, Director
Whitehorse Regional Hospital
#5, Hospital Road
Whitehorse, Yukon Y1A 3H7
(403) 667-8700 (telephone)
(403) 667-8778 (fax)

References

1. White, A., Freeth, S. and O'Brien, M. 1992: *Infant Feeding 1990*. HMSO. (A survey carried out by the Social Survey Division of the office of Population Censuses and Surveys, SS1299.)

2. Littman, H., Medendorp, S. V. and Goldfarb, J. 1994: The decision to breastfeed: the importance of fathers' approval. *Clinical Pediatrics*, vol. 33, no. 4, pp. 214-219.

3. MAIN Trial Collaborative Group 1994: Preparing for breastfeeding: treatment of inverted and non-protractile nipples in pregnancy. *Midwifery*, vol. 10, pp. 200-214.

4. Heinig, M. J., Nommsen, L. A. and Dewey, K. G. 1992: Lactation and postpartum weight loss. *Mechanisms Regulating Lactation and Infant Nutrition Utilization*, vol. 30, pp. 397-400.

5. Dewey, K. G., Heinig, M. J. and Nommsen, L. A. 1993: Maternal weight loss patterns during prolonged lactation. *Am. J. Clin. Nutr.*, vol. 58, pp. 162-166.

6. Newcomb, B. E. et al. 1994: Lactation and a reduced risk of premenopausal breast cancer. *New Engl. J. Med.*, vol. 330, no. 2, pp. 81-87.

7. UK National Case-Control Study Group 1993: Breastfeeding and risk of breast cancer in young women. *Br. Med. J.*, vol. 307, no. 6895, pp. 17-20.

8. Cancer and Steroid Hormone Study, CDC/NICHHD 1987: The reduction in risk of ovarian cancer associated with oral contraceptive use. *New Engl. J. Med.*, vol. 316, pp. 650-655.

9. Singh, K. K., Suchindran, C. M. and Singh, K. 1993: Effects of breastfeeding after resumption of menstruation on waiting time to next conception. *Human Biol.*, vol. 65, pp. 71-86.

10. Kennedy, K. I. and Visness, C. M. 1992: Contraceptive efficacy of lactational amenorrhoea. *Lancet*, vol. 339, pp. 227-230.

11. Sowers, M. et al. 1993: Changes in bone density with lactation. *J. Am. Med. Assoc.*, vol. 269, pp. 3130-3135.

12. Cummings, R. G. and Klineberg, R. J. 1993: Breastfeeding and other reproductive factors and the risk of hip fracture in elderly women. *Int. J. Epidemiol.*, vol. 2, no. 4, pp. 684-691.

13. Cockburn, F. et al. 1995: Effect of diet on the fatty acid composition of the major phospholipids of infant cerebral cortex. *Arch. Dis. Childh.*, vol. 72, pp. 198-203.

14. Makrides, M. et al. 1995: Are long-chain polyunsaturated fatty acids essential nutrients in infancy? *Lancet*, vol. 345, pp. 1463-1468.

15. Goldman, A. S. 1993: The immune system of human milk: antimicrobial, anti-inflammatory and immuno-modulating properties. *Pediatr. Infect. Dis. J.*, vol. 12, pp. 664-671.

16. Rogan, W. G. and Gladen, B. C. 1993: Breastfeeding and cognitive development. *Early Human Devel.*, vol. 31, pp. 181-193.

17. Lanting, C. I. et al. 1994: Neurological differences between nine-year-old children fed breast milk or formula milk as babies. *Lancet*, vol. 344, pp. 1319-1322.

18. Lucas, A. et al. 1992: Breast milk and subsequent intelligence quotient in children born preterm. *Lancet*, vol. 339, pp. 261-264.

19. Lucas, A. et al. 1994: A randomized multicentre study of human milk versus formula and later development in preterm infants. *Arch. Dis. Childh.*, vol. 70, no. 2, pp. F141-F146.

20. Birch, E. et al. 1993: Breastfeeding and optimal visual development. *J. Pediatr. Opthalmol. Strabismus,* vol. 30, pp. 33-38.

21. Howie, P. W. et al. 1990: Protective effect of breastfeeding against infection. *Br. Med. J.,* vol. 300, no. 6716, pp. 11-16.

22. Brock, J. 1993: Breastfeeding—the immunological case. *New Generation Digest,* no. 4, pp. 5-6.

23. Lucas, A. and Cole, T. J. 1990: Breast milk and neonatal necrotising enterocolitis. *Lancet,* vol. 336, pp. 1519-1523.

24. Burr, M. L. et al. 1993: Infant feeding, wheezing and allergy: a prospective study. *Arch. Dis. Childh.,* vol. 68, pp. 724-728.

25. Wright, L. et al. 1989: Breastfeeding and lower respiratory tract illness in the first year of life. *Br. Med. J.,* vol. 299, pp. 946-949.

26. Duncan, B. et al. 1993: Exclusive breastfeeding for at least four months protects against otitis media. *Pediatrics,* vol. 91, no. 5, pp. 867-872.

27. Aniansson, G. et al. 1994: A prospective cohort study on breastfeeding and otitis media in Swedish infants. *Pediatr. Infect. Dis. J.,* vol. 13, pp. 183-188.

28. Karajalainen, J. et al. 1992: A bovine albumin peptide as a possible trigger of insulin-dependent diabetes. *New Engl. J. Med.,* vol. 327, pp. 302-307.

29. Virtanen, S. M. et al. 1993: Early introduction of dairy products associated with increased risk of IDDM in Finnish children. *Diabetes,* vol. 42, pp. 1786-1790.

30. Monte, W. C., Johnston, C. S. and Roll, L. E. 1994: Bovine serum albumin detected in infant formula is a possible trigger for insulin-dependent diabetes mellitus. *J. Amer. Diet. Assoc.,* vol. 94, pp. 314-316.

31. Businco, L. and Cantani, A. 1990: Prevention of childhood allergy by dietary manipulation. *Clin. Exper. Allergy,* vol. 20, suppl. 3, pp. 9-14.

32. Mepham, B. 1991: Suckling-induced stimulation of breast milk. *New Generation,* vol. 10, no. 2, pp. 31-32.

33. Inch, S. and Garforth, S.: Establishing and maintaining breastfeeding. In: Chalmers, M., Enkin, M. and Keirse, M. (eds) 1989: *Effective care in pregnancy and childbirth.* Oxford Univ Pr. p. 1364.

34. Royal College of Midwives 1991: *Successful breastfeeding: a practical guide for midwives and others supporting breastfeeding mothers.* Churchill Livingstone. pp. 27-29.

35. Hey, E. 1995: Neonatal jaundice— how much do we really know? *MIDIRS Midwifery Digest,* vol. 5, no. 1, pp. 4-8.

36. De Carvalho, M. 1981: Effects of water supplementation on physiological jaundice in breastfed babies. *Arch. Dis. Childh.,* vol. 56, no. 7, pp. 568-569.

37. Beeken, S. and Waterston, T. 1992: Health service support of breastfeeding—are we practising what we preach? *Br. Med. J.,* vol. 305, pp. 285-287.

38. Welford, H. 1995: Bournemouth put breastfeeding first. *Modern Midwife,* vol. 5, no. 6, pp. 5-6.

39. Hawdon, J. M., Ward-Platt, M. P. and Aynsley-Green, A. 1992: Neonatal hypoglycaemia—blood glucose monitoring and baby feeding. *Midwifery,* vol. 9, pp. 3-6.

40. Glasier, A. S., McNeilly, A. S. and Howie, P. W. 1984: The prolactin response to suckling. *Clinical Endocrinology,* vol. 21, pp. 109-116.

41. Director General of WHO 1992: Report, EB93/17. WHO, Geneva.

42. From *Protecting, Promoting and Supporting Breastfeeding: the special role of maternity services—a joint WHO/UNICEF statement.* 1989.

43. Glazener, C. et al. Health Services Research Unit, University of Aberdeen. Main research findings forthcoming, empirical evidence submitted to the House of Commons Health Committee, January 1992. Published in the *Second Report from the Health Committee: Maternity Services (Winterton Report) 1992.* vol. 1. House of Commons Session 1991-92.

44. Whitehead, R. G. and Paul, A. A. 1984: Growth charts and the assessment of infant feeding practices in the western world and in developing countries. *Early Human Devel.,* vol. 9, pp. 187-207.

45. Dewey, K. G. et al. 1992: Growth of breastfed and formula fed infants from 0-18 months: the Darling (Davis Area Research on Lactation, Infant Nutrition and Growth) study. *Pediatrics,* vol. 89, pp. 1035-1041.

46. Gribble, G. 1995: A mother's manifesto. *New Generation,* vol. 14, no. 2, pp. 14-15.

47. See, for example, Redbridge Health Authority 1990: *Policy Statement on Breastfeeding in Public Areas of Health Authority Premises.*

48. Forsyth, J. S. et al. 1993: Relation between early introduction of solid food to infants and their weight and illnesses during the first two years of life. *Br. Med. J.,* vol. 306, pp. 1572-1576.

49. Fildes, V. 1988: *Wet nursing: a history from antiquity to the present.* Blackwell.

50. Tyson, J. E. 1977: *Nursing and prolactin secretion.* Academic Press.

51. Woolridge, M. W. et al. 1980: Effect of a traditional and of a new nipple shield on sucking patterns and milk flow. *Early Human Devel.,* vol. 4, pp. 357-362.

52. Auerback, K. G. 1990: The effect of nipple shields on maternal milk volume. *Journal of Obstetric and Neonatal Nursing,* vol. 19, no. 5, pp. 419-427.

53. Jakobsson, I. and Lindberg, T. 1983: Cow's milk proteins cause infantile colic in breastfed infants: a double-blind crossover study. *Pediatrics,* vol. 71, pp. 268-271.

54. Woolridge, M. and Fisher, C. 1988: Colic, 'overfeeding,' and symptoms of lactose malabsorption in the breastfed baby: a possible artifact of feed management? *Lancet,* no. 8605, pp. 382-384.

55. Williams, A. F. 1993: Human milk and the preterm baby. *Br. Med. J.,* vol. 306, pp. 1628-1629.

56. Williams, A. F. 1994: Is breastfeeding beneficial in the UK? Statement of the Standing Committee on Nutrition of the British Pediatric Association. *Arch. Dis. Childh.,* vol. 71, pp. 376-380.

57. Howie, P. et al. 1980: The relationship between suckling induced prolactin metabolism. *J. Clin. Endocrinol Metab.,* vol. 50, pp. 670-673.

58. Howie, P. 1985: Breastfeeding—a new understanding. *Midwives Chronicle,* July, pp. 184-192.

59. Jones, E. 1994: Breastfeeding in the preterm infant. *Modern Midwife,* vol. 4, no. 1, pp. 22-26.

60. DeCarvalho, M. et al. 1985: frequency of milk expression and milk production by mothers of non-nursing premature neonates. *AJDC,* vol. 139, pp. 483-485.

61. Minchin, M. 1987: Premature babies: why breast is best. *New Generation,* vol. 6, no. 3, pp. 36-37.

62. Palmer, G. 1993: Any old iron? *Health Visitor,* vol. 66, no. 7, pp. 248-249, 252.

Index

Index

.... *231*

Other fine pregnancy and childcare titles you'll want to have and enjoy, available at fine bookstores near you . . .

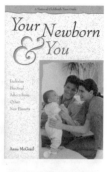
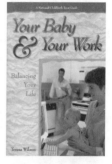
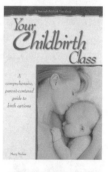
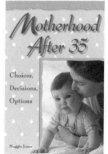

. . .our best-selling "Your Pregnancy" series. . .

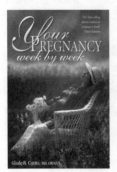

$12.95 • ISBN 1-55561-143-5
6 x 9¼, 384 pages, illustrated, paperback

Your Pregnancy Week by Week
Third Edition

Glade B. Curtis, MD, OB/GYN

Completely updated in its third edition, *Your Pregnancy Week by Week* is the top-selling pregnancy book written by a doctor. Dr. Curtis designed its unique format to help all women from before they conceive their baby until they give birth. Learn how your baby is developing and review changes in your own body as they happen. A vast amount of invaluable information about the entire pregnancy is included.

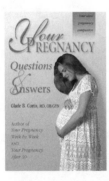

$12.95 • ISBN 1-55561-150-8
6 x 9¼, 432 pages, illustrated, paperback

Your Pregnancy Questions & Answers

Glade B. Curtis, MD, OB/GYN

This bestseller is in an easy-to-read question-and-answer format. Dr. Curtis thoughtfully answers more than 1,200 questions pregnant women ask most often. Includes questions you worry about but may feel are "not important enough to bother my doctor," or are too personal to discuss.

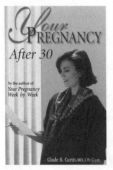

$12.95 • ISBN 1-55561-088-9
6 x 9¼, 384 pages, illustrated, paperback

Your Pregnancy After 30

Glade B. Curtis, MD, OB/GYN

The latest in this best-selling series—an important and timely resource for the rapidly growing number of women becoming pregnant after age 30. Covers: achieving pregnancy after 30, multiple births, managing fatigue, tests for baby and mother, nutrition and weight management and workplace safety.

visit our website at www.fisherbooks.com

. . .popular, illustrated guides in full color throughout. . .

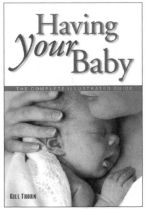

$15.95 • ISBN 1-55561-133-8
6¼ x 9, 208 pages, 93 color photographs,
34 color illustrations, paperback

Having Your Baby
The Complete Illustrated Guide
Gill Thorn

Packed with clear explanations, sound advice and color illustrations, *Having Your Baby* covers the questions and issues a pregnant woman and her partner need to know, including:

- Pre-conception health and pregnancy planning
- How your growing baby develops month by month
- Self-care tips for good nutrition, exercise, sleeping better, and more
- Your relationship with your partner
- Choices for prenatal care
- Where to have your baby
- Labor and birth
- Getting to know your newborn

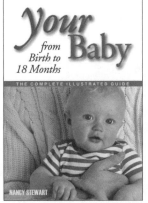

$15.95 • ISBN 1-55561-134-6
6¼ x 9, 192 pages, 81 color photographs,
27 color illustrations, paperback

Your Baby from Birth to 18 Months
The Complete Illustrated Guide
Nancy Stewart

Here is all the information and reassurance new parents are likely to need, from the birth of their baby to 18 months old. This practical illustrated guide to baby care covers:

- Settling in during the first few weeks
- Feeding—both breast- and bottlefeeding, weaning and solid foods
- Diaper changing
- Bathing your baby
- Your child's physical, intellectual and emotional development
- Getting your baby to sleep
- Coping with excessive crying
- Health matters and safety in the home

visit our website at www.fisherbooks.com

...excellent, easy-to-read information for first-time mothers...

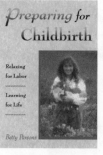

$9.95 • ISBN 1-55561-128-1
6 x 9, 144 pages, illustrated, paperback

Preparing for Childbirth
Relaxing for Labor ~ Learning for Life
Betty Parsons

A voice pregnant women will listen to—encouraging, witty, understanding, calm. During her long career, Betty Parsons has coached more than 20,000 women through childbirth.

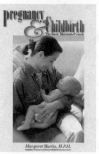

$9.95 • ISBN 1-55561-114-1
7 x 10, 128 pages, fully illustrated in two colors, paperback

Pregnancy & Childbirth
The Basic Illustrated Guide
Margaret Martin, M.P.H.

For pregnant women and their families, a conception-to-birth guide to pregnancy—written in clear, easy-to-understand terms, with informative two-color illustrations on almost every page.

...also available in Spanish...

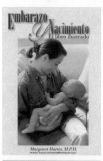

$9.95 • ISBN 1-55561-135-4
7 x 10, 128 pages, fully illustrated in two colors, paperback

Embarazo y Nacimiento
El libro ilustrado
Margaret Martin, M.P.H.

The Spanish version of our popular *Pregnancy & Childbirth*. Written in clear, easy-to-understand terms, with informative two-color illustrations on almost every page.

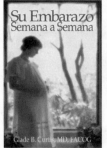

$12.95 • ISBN 1-55561-061-7
6 x 9, 436 pages, illustrated, paperback

Su Embarazo Semana a Semana
Glade B. Curtis, MD, OB/GYN

Our best-selling *Your Pregnancy Week by Week* is also available in this Spanish-language edition.

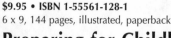